Machine Learning in Medicine

Ton J. Cleophas • Aeilko H. Zwinderman

Machine Learning in Medicine

Part Three

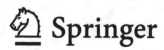
Springer

Ton J. Cleophas
Department Medicine
Albert Schweitzer Hospital
Sliedrecht, The Netherlands

Aeilko H. Zwinderman
Department Biostatistics and Epidemiology
Academic Medical Center
Amsterdam, The Netherlands

Additional material to this book can be downloaded from extras.springer.com

ISBN 978-94-024-0260-5   ISBN 978-94-007-7869-6 (eBook)
DOI 10.1007/978-94-007-7869-6
Springer Dordrecht Heidelberg New York London

Printed on acid-free paper

Springer is part of Springer Science+Business Media (www.springer.com)

Machine Learning in Medicine Part Three

by

TON J. CLEOPHAS, MD, PhD, Professor,
Past-President American College of Angiology,
Co-Chair Module Statistics Applied to Clinical Trials,
European Interuniversity College of Pharmaceutical Medicine, Lyon, France,
Department Medicine, Albert Schweitzer Hospital, Dordrecht, Netherlands

AEILKO H. ZWINDERMAN, MathD, PhD, Professor,
President International Society of Biostatistics,
Co-Chair Module Statistics Applied to Clinical Trials,
European Interuniversity College of Pharmaceutical Medicine, Lyon, France,
Department Biostatistics and Epidemiology, Academic Medical Center, Amsterdam,
Netherlands

With the help from

HENNY I. CLEOPHAS-ALLERS, BChem

Preface

Machine learning is a novel discipline for data analysis that started some 40 years ago with the advent of the computer. It is already widely implemented in socio-/econometry, but not so in medicine, probably due to the traditional belief of clinicians in clinical trials where the effects of multiple variables tend to even out by the randomization process and are not further taken into account. Machine learning is different from traditional data analysis, because, unlike means and standard deviations, it uses proximities between data, data patterns, pattern recognition, data thresholding and data trafficking. It is more flexible than traditional statistical methods, and it can process big data and hundreds of variables, and data, for which analysis without the help of a computer would be impossible.

This does not mean that the mathematics of machine learning is simple. Often integrals, derivatives, complex matrices and other calculus methods, as developed in the seventeenth century by great western mathematicians like Newton and Leibnitz, are applied. It is gratifying to observe, that, three centuries later, mathematicians from the same schools are responsible for the founding of important machine learning methodologies.

The first two parts of this volume reviewed basic machine learning methods like, *cluster analysis, neural networks, factor analysis, Bayesian networks and support vector machines*. The current Part Three of this volume assesses more recent and more advanced methods such as the ones described underneath:

Newton's methods, as the most advanced methods for fitting experimental data to a mathematical prediction function.

Stochastic methods, including advanced Markov modeling, adjusted for irreversible complications and death.

Complex sampling, for obtaining unbiased samples from big demographic data.

Optimal binning, for advanced classification learning of health and health-education parameters.

Evolutionary operations, for advanced search of optimal solutions to many scientific questions, including evolutionary algorithms, neuroevolution, genetic programming, and genetic algorithms.

Each chapter of the current book was written in a way much similar to that of the first two volumes, and

1. Will describe a novel method that has already been successfully applied in the authors' own research
2. Will provide the analysis of medical data examples
3. Will provide step-by-step analyses for the benefit of the readers
4. Will provide the commands to be given to the software programs applied (mostly SPSS)
5. Can be studied without the need to consult other chapters
6. Will be written in a explanatory way for a readership of mainly non-mathematicians
7. Will be provided together with a data file on the internet through extras.springer.com for the benefit of investigators who wish to perform their own analyses

We should add that the authors are well-qualified in their field. Professor Zwinderman is president of the International Society of Biostatistics (2012–2015), and Prof. Cleophas is past-president of the American College of Angiology (2000–2002). From their expertise they should be able to make adequate selections of modern methods for clinical data analysis for the benefit of physicians, students, and investigators. The authors have been working and publishing together for 15 years, and their research can be characterized as a continued effort to demonstrate that clinical data analysis is not mathematics but rather a discipline at the interface of biology and mathematics.

The authors as professors and teachers in statistics for 20 years are convinced that the current part three of this three-volume book contains information unpublished so far and vital to the analysis of the complex medical data as commonly witnessed today.

Machine learning is a novel discipline concerned with the analysis of large data and multiple variables. It involves computationally intensive methods, and is currently mainly the domain of computer scientists, and is already commonly used in social sciences, marketing research, operational research and applied sciences.

Machine learning is virtually unused in clinical research. This is probably due to the traditional belief of clinicians in clinical trials where multiple variables are equally balanced by the randomization process and are not further taken into account. In contrast, modern computer data files often involve hundreds of variables like genes and other laboratory values, and computationally intensive methods are required for their analysis.

Lyon, France   Ton J. Cleophas
02-09-2013   Aeilko H. Zwinderman

Contents

Contents of Machine Learning in Medicine Part One

Contents of Machine Learning in Medicine Part Two

Chapter 1
Introduction to Machine Learning in Medicine Part Three

1 Summary

1.1 Objective

This chapter summarizes the different machine learning methodologies reviewed in the 60 chapters of this 3 volume book.

1.2 Results and Conclusions

1. Machine learning is different from traditional data analysis, because, unlike means and standard deviations, it uses proximities between data, data patterns, pattern recognition, data thresholding and data trafficking.
2. The first two parts of this volume reviewed basic machine learning methods like, *cluster analysis, neural networks, factor analysis, Bayesian networks and support vector machines.*
3. The current part three of this volume assesses more recent and more advanced methods, including *Newton's methods, stochastic methods, complex sampling, optimal binning, evolutionary operations.*

2 Introduction

Machine learning is a novel discipline for data analysis that started some 40 years ago with the advent of the computer. It is already widely implemented in socio-/econometry, but not so in medicine, probably due to the traditional belief of clinicians in clinical trials where the effects of multiple variables tend to even out by the randomization process and are not further taken into account. Machine

T.J. Cleophas and A.H. Zwinderman, *Machine Learning in Medicine: Part Three*,
DOI 10.1007/978-94-007-7869-6_1, © Springer Science+Business Media Dordrecht 2013

learning is different from traditional data analysis, because, unlike means and standard deviations, it uses proximities between data, data patterns, pattern recognition, data thresholding and data trafficking. It is more flexible than traditional statistical methods, and it can process big data and hundreds of variables, and data, for which analysis without the help of a computer would be impossible. In this introductory chapter we will summarize the methods reviewed in the 60 chapters of this 3 volume book entitled Machine Learning in Medicine. Stepwise analyses will be given per chapter, this chapter contains a succinct description of the practical use and relevance to the medical community of the new methods, and we will briefly mention the limitations of the traditional methods used so far.

3   Contents of Part One of This 3 Volume Book

Machine learning can be defined as knowledge for making predictions as obtained from processing training data through a computer. Because data sets often involve multiple variables, data analyses are complex and modern computationally intensive methods have to be used for the purpose. The first part of the current 3 volume book reviewed important methods relevant for health care and research, although little used in the field of medicine so far.

1. Logistic Regression for Health Profiling

    One of the first machine learning methods used in health research is logistic regression for health profiling where single combinations of x-variables are used to predict the risk of a medical event in single persons (Chap. 2).

2. Optimal Scaling Discretization
    Optimal Scaling Regularization

    A wonderful method for analyzing imperfect data with multiple variables is optimal scaling (Chaps. 3 and 4).

3. Partial Correlations

    Partial correlations analysis is the best method for removing interaction effects from large clinical datasets (Chap. 5).

4. Mixed Linear Modeling
    Binary Partitioning
    Item Response Modeling
    Time Dependent Predictor Modeling
    Seasonality Assessments

    Mixed linear modeling (1), binary partitioning (2), item response modeling (3), time dependent predictor analysis (4) and autocorrelation (5) are linear or loglinear regression methods suitable for assessing data with respectively repeated measures (1), binary decision trees (2), exponential exposure-response relationships (3), different values at different periods (4) and those with seasonal differences (5), (Chaps. 6, 7, 8, 9, and 10).

5. Non-linear Modeling
    Multilayer Perceptron Modeling
    Radial Basis Function Modeling

Clinical data sets with non-linear relationships between exposure and outcome variables require special analysis methods, and can usually also be adequately analyzed with neural network methods like multilayer perceptron networks, and radial basis function networks (Chaps. 11, 12, and 13).

6. Factor Analysis
    Hierarchical Cluster Analysis (Unsupervised Machine Learning)

Clinical data with multiple exposure variables are usually analyzed using analysis of (co-) variance (AN(C)OVA), but this method does not adequately account the relative importance of the variables and their interactions. Factor analysis and hierarchical cluster analysis account for all of these limitations (Chaps. 14 and 15).

7. Partial Least Squares
    Discriminant Analysis (Supervised Machine Learning)
    Canonical Regression

Data with multiple outcome variables are usually analyzed with multivariate analysis of (co-) variance (MAN(C)OVA). However, this has the same limitations as ANOVA. Partial least squares analysis, discriminant analysis, and canonical regression account all of these limitations (Chaps. 16, 17, and 18).

8. Fuzzy Modeling

Fuzzy modeling is a method suitable for modeling soft data, like data that are partially true or response patterns that are different at different times (Chap. 19).

4 Contents of Part Two of This 3 Volume Book

Already prior to the completion of the first volume the authors came to realize that additional methods accounting the effects of potential biases of the reported methods were available. Also, some of the methods not reported so far might provide better fit for some clinical data sets. These points were the main reasons for writing the book "Machine Learning in Medicine Part Two".

1. Two-stage Least Squares
    Quality of life Assessments with Odds Ratios
    Logistic Regression for Assessing Novel Diagnostic Tests against Control
    Association Rule Learning
    Support Vector Machines

First, we reviewed methods that are more sensitive than traditional methods, e.g., multistage least square as compared to traditional least squares (Chap. 2), logistic regression with the odds of disease as outcome as compared to concordance statistics (Chap. 6), association rule learning as compared to simple regression (Chap. 11), the odds ratio approach to quality of life for better precision than that of traditional summation of scores (Chap. 5), support vector machines for modeling dependent variables with better sensitivity/specificity than traditional logistic regression (Chap. 15).

2. Multiple Imputations
   Two-dimensional Clustering
   Multidimensional Clustering
   Anomaly Detection
   Correspondence Analysis
   Multivariate Analysis of Time Series
   Bayesian Networks

Second, we reviewed methods that are extensions of traditional methods, like two-dimensional (Chap. 8) and multidimensional clustering (Chap. 9), support vector machines (Chap. 15), anomaly detections (Chap. 10), that can be considered as extensions of simple hierarchical clustering (Chap. 15 vol 1). Also correspondence analysis (Chap. 13) is a 3×3 (or more) extension of simple 2×2 contingency table analysis. Autoregressive integrated moving average (ARIMA) (Chap. 14) is an extension of simple autocorrelations (Chap. 10 vol 1), and so is discrete wavelet analysis of continuous wavelet analysis (Chap. 19), multiple imputations of the more simple methods of dealing with missing data like regression imputation (Chap. 3), Bayesian networks of more basic regression models for causal relationships (Chap. 16).

3. Bhattacharya Modeling
   Validating Surrogate Endpoints
   Multidimensional Scaling
   Protein and DNA Sequence Mining
   Continuous Sequential Techniques

Third, we reviewed methods for which there is no alternative, like multidimensional scaling for assessing patients' personal meanings (Chap. 12), validating surrogate endpoints (Chap. 7), Bhattacharya modeling for finding hidden Gaussian subgroups in large populations (Chap. 4), continuous sequential techniques (Chap. 18), string/sequence mining of very large data (Chap. 17).

4. Bhattacharya Modeling
   Two-dimensional Clustering
   Multidimensional Clustering
   Anomaly Detection
   Multidimensional Scaling

We added that, unlike traditional statistical methods, many machine learning methodologies consist of so-called unsupervised data, i.e., datasets without outcome variables. Instead of classification of the data according to their outcome values, the data are, then, classified according to their proximity, entropy, density, pattern. The Chaps. 4, 8, 9, 10, and 12 are examples.

5 Contents of Part Three of This 3 Volume Book

1. Evolutionary Operations

The current third part of this 3 volume book starts with the very modern analytical method of evolutionary operations (Chap. 2). No other field in medical research involves more variables than genome wide data files. The human genome consists of about 20,500 genes and all of these genes are potential predictor variables of health and disease. At random subsets of genes are selected and differences between optimal prediction of a disease and observed prediction, using, e.g., the magnitudes of correlation coefficients are applied to define the goodness of fit of the subsets as predictors of a disease. Iterations and breedings of the subset genes (generation after generation) appear to enhance the chance of finding subsets of genes with excellent fit. All this sounds pretty abstract, but it works well, even with a data file of 20,000 variables. After 80 generations or so the data may converse and no better fit is found anymore. A pleasant thing about genetic operations is that it works well, not only with genetic data, but also with any type of data with many variables. The 500 patient study of Vinterbo who used subsets from 43 predictor variables, e.g., correctly predicted the risk of myocardial infarction after 79 generations [1]. Evolutionary operations are now applied in many fields like genetic programming for finding the best computer program for its purpose, or neuroevolutionary planning for finding the best neural network for its purpose.

2. Multiple Treatments, Multiple Endpoints

The problem with big data involving many variables deserves full attention with machine learning, because of increased risks of type I errors of finding differences by chance, and the Chaps. 3 and 4 review standard and novel methods for the purpose. Unfortunately, multiple comparison adjustments are not always appropriately taken into account in machine learning software, and investigators may need to perform adjustments on their own part. On the other hand, the multiple testing problem is largest in data where any variable may have a strong probability of being an important predictor. In many situations like with genome studies, it is rightly assumed that only one or two variables have strong probabilities, among others with a probability of virtually zero. Yet, type I errors may occur even with two statistical tests, and should be accounted even so.

3. Optimal Binning

The Chap. 5 addresses optimal binning. Modern clinical data files are usually big and data analysis is correspondingly laborious, requiring much computer memory, sometimes even more than a standard personal computer can offer. An important function of machine learning methodologies is to find methods for data analysis that use fewer numerical data without loss of information. One of the ways of obtaining this is optimal binning, where, essentially, continuous variables are discretized into discrete variables, in such a way, that all the relevant information is maintained or even improved, and yet less computer memory is needed.

4. Exact P-values

The Chap. 6 addresses exact p-values. Traditionally, a p-value represents the probability of no effect in your data and is expressed as $<$ some percentage, e.g., <5 %. However, modern software uses very precise statistical tables and can produce p-values like 0.067 or 0.004. These p-values are, then, interpreted as core criteria for making decisions about the approximate risk one is willing to take. Particularly, the term "approximate" should be emphasized, because p-values are only entirely-true, if calculated from random samples, and big observational data are mostly un-random, minimizing the robustness of the calculated p-values. Yet the scientific community is very familiar with p-values, and also in machine learning they are often applied, although more often as criterion for decision making than as measure for no effect in the data.

5. Probit Regression

Multiple outcomes research of events is very common with big clinical data, like demographic data and post marketing surveillance data. Multivariate probit regression appeared here to be a better tool for analysis than traditional multivariate logistic regression. It is not available in SPSS [2], but the probit module in STATA [3] works fine. The Chap. 7 gives an example of multivariate probit regression of a clinical data example.

6. Over-dispersion

Already in the Chaps. 3 and 4 of the first issue of this 3 volume book the problem of over-dispersion was addressed, particularly in connection with data discretization, meaning that continuous data are categorized or rescaled. The consequence is often, that the computed standard errors are wider than compatible with Gaussian modeling, and that some kind of regularization of the standard errors is desirable, before Gaussian statistics can be performed. The Chap. 8 gives rules and procedures to adjust over-dispersion.

7. Random Effects Modeling

Random effects are unexpected effects. Generally speaking, the bigger the data, the more chance that such effects will be observed. In the event of random effects, the spread in the data is mainly caused, not by the residues in the data, but by the random effects themselves. Special data analysis methods are required. Chapter 9 gives several examples of such effects in clinical data sets, and gives their analyses.

8. Weighted Least Squares

Linear regression is the traditional tool for the analysis of multiple exposure variables, like treatment modalities, age, gender, co-morbidities and co-medications and other patient characteristics. The problem is that linear regression assumes that the spread in the outcome data is equal for each value of the exposure variable. This assumption is not warranted in many real life situations. This point, particularly, applies to the big data obtained from demographic data or surveys. Weighted least squares is the solution if the assumption of equal spread is not warranted. Examples and step-by-step analyses are given in Chap. 10.

9. Multiple Response Sets

The Chap. 11 addresses multiple response sets. Machine learning can better describe detailed clinical data than traditional methods do. E.g., detailed clinical data often involve related qualitative questions about a single underlying disease. Traditional summary statistics would tell us something about each question separately. An example is given.

Of 3,034 patients visiting their doctor 811 answered a question about ill feeling		
traditional analysis	391 yes-answers	(43.3 %)
multiple response analysis	391	(12.9 %).

The 12.9 % is the percentage of all yes answers as given to all (9) questions, while the 43.3 % is the percentage of yes answers to a single question. The magnitude of the first percentage, unlike that of the second, tells us something about the impact of the question in relation with the other 8 questions. This is relevant, because, together, they present the burden of a doctor's outpatient clinic.

10. Complex Samples

The research of entire populations is costly and obtaining information from selected samples instead is more time- and cost-efficient. However, the latter method is generally biased due to selection bias. Complex sample technology adjusts for selection bias by assigning appropriate weights to each individual included. It is better suitable for the research of entire populations than selected samples, and provides unbiased subsamples from demographic data. Chapter 12 reviews the methodology and gives data examples.

11. Runs Test

R square values (squared correlation coefficients) are traditionally used for finding the best fit mathematical model to describe clinical data sets. However, r-square values are not very sensitive, and pretty large r-squares may still indicate a poor data fit. The runs test is a simple alternative that, generally, performs better for the purpose. Chapter 13 compares the two approaches and confirms the better performance of the runs test.

12. Decision Trees

Decision trees are a fundamental methodology for decision analyses of real world problems. They assess the effects of predictor variables on numbers of events and other health outcomes, like continuous health outcomes. In SPSS statistical software (1) the chi-square automatic interaction detection (CHAID) and (2) the continuous outcome tree analyses (CRT) are available. Chapter 14 reviews both methods, and explains them with the help of data examples, that are analyzed in a stepwise way.

13. Spectral Plots

Time series often show many peaks and irregular spaces in between. Autocorrelation is a standard analysis method (Chap. 10 vol 1). However, it is not very sensitive with many irregularities in the data. Chapter 15 reviews spectral plots, a very sophisticated method for analyzing time series with a lot of irregularities. It is based on periodograms with frequency on the x- and amplitude on the y-axis, as obtained from Fourier modeling. A comparison is given with autocorrelation modeling.

14. Newton's Methods

Isaac Newton (1711)'s methods determine the best fit mathematical function for a data set just like regression methods, but unlike regression methods they make no selection for a specific function pattern, like exponential or quadratic function pattern, but include many types of mathematical functions in a simultaneous modeling program. Newton's methods are re-discovered in the past two decades, and are, currently, considered the most advanced way of fitting non-linear data. Chapter 16 reviews the methods, and uses pharmacodynamic/-kinetic data for the purpose.

15. Stochastic Processes

The Chaps. 17 and 18 review stationary and absorbing Markov chains, suitable for long term predictions from short term population surveys. The stationary ones predict reversible nonfatal diseases, the absorbing ones predict irreversible complications and death. Stochastic processes are very popular machine learning tools, but predictions are far beyond the interval of observation, and, therefore, predictions may not be correct. Nonetheless, the methodology is precious, because, although it does not show the future, it does show what will happen, if nothing changes.

16. Conjoint Analysis

The Chap. 19 reviews conjoint analysis, a machine learning method for assessing interactions in the data without the need to add interaction terms to the data. The problem with traditional methods for assessing interaction between predictor variables like ANOVA (analysis of variance) and regression methods, is, that interaction terms have to be added to the data and that only one or two interaction terms are possible, because, otherwise, statistical power will rapidly be lost. This is not the case with conjoint analysis, and it is a pleasant method, particularly in data sets with plenty of interactions, like big observational machine learning data files.

6 Conclusions

1. Machine learning is different from traditional data analysis, because, unlike means and standard deviations, it uses proximities between data, data patterns, pattern recognition, data thresholding and data trafficking.
2. The first two parts of this volume reviewed basic machine learning methods like, *cluster analysis, neural networks, factor analysis, Bayesian networks and support vector machines.*
3. The current part three of this volume assesses more recent and more advanced methods, including *Newton's methods, stochastic methods, complex sampling, optimal binning, evolutionary operations.*

References

1. Vinterbo S, Ohno L (1999) A genetic algorithm to select variables in logistic regression: example in the domain of myocardial infarction. In: Proceedings of the AMIA (American Medical Information Association) symposium 1999, Washington, DC, USA, pp 984–988
2. SPSS Statistical Software (2013) www.spss.com. 09 Aug 2013
3. STATA Statistical Software (2013) www.stata.com. 09 Aug 2013

Chapter 2
Evolutionary Operations

1 Summary

1.1 Background

Evolutionary operations are sets of rules based on biological evolution mechanisms like mutation, recombination, and selection, and are, sometimes, used to analyze data files with thousands of variables like genes.

1.2 Objective

To test whether they can be effectively used in patients with Marfan syndrome for the identification from the entire pool of genes of the human genome a subset of genes strongly associated with a large aorta.

1.3 Methods

In 55 patients with Marfan syndrome a genome wide study was performed. Affymetrix exon chips were used using RNA from skin biopsies. The R Package *Subselections* was applied for analysis.

1.4 Results

Evolutionary operations were effective to identify a subset of genes discriminating between patients with large and small aortas at $p < 0.0001$. A standard logistic

T.J. Cleophas and A.H. Zwinderman, *Machine Learning in Medicine: Part Three*,
DOI 10.1007/978-94-007-7869-6_2, © Springer Science+Business Media Dordrecht 2013

regression of the best fit genes produced a multiple correlation coefficient of 0.878, indicating that the selected genes were very good predictors of large aortas.

1.5   Conclusions

1. Evolutionary operations are sets of rules based on biological evolution mechanisms like gene mutation and recombination, and selection of the fittest subjects.
2. They are used for finding best fit models and subsets, and are useful and effective in data with many variables.
3. They do not use prior distribution functions, and no guarantee can be given that an optimal function or subset is found.
4. Solutions should be tested against the results from traditional analysis methods like regression models.
5. In our example of 55 patients with Marfan syndrome evolutionary operations were effective to identify a subset of genes discriminating between patients with large and small aortas.
6. Evolutionary operations is adequate even if there are thousands of variables like genes.

2   Introduction

Evolutionary algorithms [1] are optimization algorithms that are based on mechanisms inspired by biological evolution such as mutation, recombination and selection. These algorithms are normally used in high-dimensional spaces with thousands of variables and they do well, because the algorithms do not use assumptions on the shape of the criterion-function that is to be optimized. There is however no guarantee, that an evolutionary algorithm finds the optimum, and therefore they are especially useful, when an approximate solution is acceptable. There are many machine learning techniques that use similar evolutionary operations. Among these are (1) genetic programming to search for the best computer program, (2) neuroevolution to search for the best neural networks, and (3) genetic algorithms to search for the best subset of variables. In this chapter we will focus on genetic algorithms, but the principles apply to other applications areas as well. Genetic algorithms are key algorithms in artificial intelligence, that are used in many scientific fields to find optimal solutions. Examples are code-breaking, robotics, linguistic analysis, protein folding, and gene expression profiling. As an example, we will use genetic algorithms to find the optimal set of genes whose expression best discriminates between 55 patients with Marfan syndrome with severe or mild aortic phenotype. The R Package *Subselect* was used for data analysis [2].

Table 2.1 Characteristics of patients with small (≤47 mm) and large (>47 mm) aortic root diameters

	Patients with small diameters (n = 29)	Patients with large diameters (n = 26)
Age (years): mean (SD)	39 (10)	30 (12)
Body Surface Area (m²): mean (SD)	2.00 (0.25)	2.05 (0.24)
Male gender: n(%)	10 (35 %)	19 (73 %)

3 Example Data

The data that we use to illustrate genetic algorithms comes from a clinical trial of patients with Marfan syndrome (MFS) [3]. This syndrome is clinically defined, but is, genetically, assumed to be caused by mutations in the fibrillin gene or related genes. The syndrome has several physiological and anatomical phenotypes, but a potentially lethal complication is the development of thoracal aortic aneurysms, especially in the aortic root, which may dissect or rupture. There is large variation between MFS patients with respect to the growth-rate of the aortic diameters. To find biomarkers of fast growing aortic roots, genome wide gene expression was measured in skin biopsies of 55 patients that were included in a clinical trial evaluating the efficacy of an angiotensin II receptor antagonist to reduce the aortic growth rate. Baseline aortic root diameters were measured with echocardiography. Gene expression was measured with the Affymetrix exon chip using RNA derived from whole skin biopsies taken at the same time as that of the measurement of the aortic root diameter. Some patient characteristics are reported in Table 2.1. Gene expression levels of 18,072 genes were univariately associated with aortic root diameters. After multiple test correction we found that 43 genes (p < 0.000001) were significantly associated with aortic root diameters. Secondary aim was to find a set of multiple genes whose expression values best discriminated between patients with larger or smaller aortas. We used a genetic algorithm to find the optimal set of genes.

4 Methodological Background of Genetic Algorithms

The aim to find a subset of variables that best discriminates between two subgroups of patients is a well known problem in biomedical research. Although there are many valid arguments against variable-selection algorithms, it is absolutely impossible to estimate a reliable prediction model with 18,072 predictor variables with only 55 observations. So, some sort of variable selection is necessary in the present example. There are many variable selection algorithms. Well known algorithms are the stepwise forward and stepwise backward algorithms, but both have the drawback that only a small subset of all possible combinations of predictor variables are considered. Actually, if there are k predictor variables, only k possible subsets are (maximally) evaluated by the stepwise methods. An alternative variable selection algorithm considers all possible k! subsets (i.e. factorial(k)). With k = 18,072 predictor variables, there are uncountable many possible subsets. Of course, one would never consider more than, say, m = 5 predictor variables, but the number of different subsets of m predictor variables out of a total of k predictor variables is

$$\binom{k}{m},$$

and if k = 18,072 and m = 5 the number of possible subsets is

$$\binom{18,072}{5} = 10^{36}$$

It is impossible to evaluate the discriminatory ability of all those subsets. Genetic algorithms are used to search to the best subset.

The genetic algorithm first requires a function that is to be optimized. In our example the primary aim is to discriminate between MFS patient with small or large aortas. Different statistical regression models and machine learning tools may be used for discrimination between these subgroups of patients, such as logistic or tree regression analysis, random forests, neural networks, or support vector machines. Here, we will use standard logistic regression analysis. With such logistic regression model we estimate for each patient the probability, p, that he/she will have a large aorta and this probability is calculated as a function of the expression levels of the patient on the selected genes. The logistic regression model discriminates well if the observed outcome y_i of patient i (a large or a small aorta) is close to the predicted outcome p_i. The function to be optimized is therefore a function F of the summed differences

$$F = \sum \left(|y_i - p_i| \right)^r,$$

where r is usually chosen as r = 1 or r = 2. The subset(s) of variables that minimize(s) this function F is(are) found by an iterative process.

1. First, a large number of subsets of between 1 and m predictor variables is selected at random and F is calculated for all subsets. A subset consists of two subsubsets that mimick the pairs of two chromosomes of a human gene. If we accept at most m = 10 predictor variables in a subset, a possible subset may be the combination of two subsubsets of predictor variables numbers, for instance, (1,2,3,4,5) and (588,3478,10774,13726,14851). Another combination may be the subsubsets of predictor variables (2051,5279,16008,16520,17718) and (1322,4348,8457,11599,152040).

2. From these initial subsets the next generation of subsets is derived by combining subsubsets of pairs of the initial subsets: i.e. the parents. The pairing is

however subject to "natural selection". Subsets of predictor variables with lower F-values are more likely to "breed" a new generation of subsets than subsets with larger F-values. It is also possible to derive the new generation from combining more than two parents and there is substantial evidence that combining more parents produce better offspring. So, if we combine the parent with the two subsubsets (1,2,3,4,5) and (588,3478,10774,13726,14851) with the parent with subsubsets (2051,5279,16008,16520,17718) and (1322,4348,8457,11599,152040), a child may be generated with subsubsets (1,2,3,4,5) and (1322,4348,8457,11599,152040). Other "genetic" operations, such as drift, extinction and migration, may be used as well to produce a new generation.

3. The process of breeding a new generation may be subject to "mutation" and "recombination". Mutation refers to the possibility that a predictor variables in a subsubset is substituted by another predictor variable. Thus, the subsubset of predictor variables numbers (1322,4348,8457,11599,152040) from the second parent may be changed into the subset (1322,4348,88,11599,152040) by substituting predictor variable 8457 by predictor variable 88. Mutations may also concern the change of multiple predictor variables in a subsubset or deletions or insertions of one or more predictor variables to the subsubset. Recombination refers to the exchange of predictor variables from a subsubset of a parent to the other subsubset of this parent . If the parent subsets are (1,2,3,4,5) and (588,3478,10774,13726,14851), an offspring may have subsubset (1,2,3,13726,14851) from parent 1 and (1322,4348,88,11599,152040) from parent 2 (including the mutation).

4. For all subsets in the new generation the function F will have to be calculated.

The iterative process can be terminated by hand, after a fixed number of generations, after fixed computing time, or, if new subsets in new generations do not further improve the objective function F. Crucial tuning parameters are the probabilities of mutation and recombination. There are, unfortunately, no practical guidelines to choose upper and lower boundaries for these probabilities.

Genetic algorithms are easy to program, but it is not well understood why genetic algorithms work well in many applications. The genetic heuristics provide only weak indications for the search-direction for the best subset of predictor variables, so genetic algorithms are only marginally better than full random searching. Limiting factors for the efficiency of genetic algorithms are the repeated evaluation of the objective function F (which may be time-consuming) and the complexity of the objective function. Modeling a human cell from all the constituting organelles , proteins, DNA and RNA molecules is much too complex. The same applies to designing a plane or a house. Genetic algorithms also have the tendency to converge to a local optimum rather than the global optimum. This may be investigated by running the algorithm multiple times and by varying the mutation and recombination rates.

Several software packages provide genetic algorithms for variable selection. The package *Subselect* in the R program [2] offers genetic algorithms as one alternative and allows comparison with complete search, simulated annealing, and restrictive improvement. Other R-packages offer stepwise selection algorithms and bootstrap-based approaches.

5   Results of a Genetic Algorithm to Variable Selection in Our Example Data

We used the implementation of the genetic algorithm in the R-package *Subselect* [2]. The distribution of the univariate correlations of the expression-levels of each gene with aortic diameter is illustrated in Fig. 2.1a. Out of 18,072 correlations, there were 4,853 with p-values <0.05 and 43 with p-values $<10^{-6}$. Largest univariate correlation was 0.54. For the multiple regression model, the genetic algorithm was allowed to select maximally 10 genes. From Fig. 2.1b it becomes clear that there were many subsets of 10 predictor variables with very similar multiple correlation coefficients. The best subset of 10 predictor variables had multiple correlation coefficient of 0.893. Standard forward stepwise regression analysis until 10 predictor variables were selected, yielded multiple correlation coefficient of 0.878.

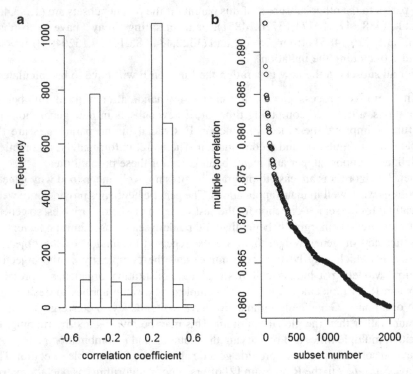

Fig. 2.1 Univariate correlations between gene-expression levels and aortic diameter size (**a**), multiple correlation between a subset of gene-expression levels and aortic diameter size (**b**)

6 Discussion

Genetic algorithms are useful tools for biomedical researchers. The heuristic operations derived from biological evolution and molecular genetics have proven to be effective in optimizing mathematical-statistical functions too. It cannot however be guaranteed that genetic algorithms actually find the global optimum (if it exists), and therefore solutions should be compared with results from other algorithms.

Evolutionary operations are convenient, e.g., to genetic programming, neuroevolution, and genetic algorithms. They are respectively used for finding the computer programs, neural networks, and subset of genes with the best sensitivity, reliability and precision to be health and disease. Evolutionary operations are, however, also convenient for the selection of the best subsets of any other data file with multiple predictor variables. As an example Vinterbo et al. [4] used it in a study of 500 patients with chest pain and 43 predictor variables. After 79 generations the best fit model was selected, meaning the model with the smallest difference between the observed and predicted outcome.

7 Conclusions

1. Evolutionary operations are sets of rules based on biological evolution mechanisms like gene mutation and recombination, and the selection of the fittest subjects.
2. They are used for finding best fit models and subsets, and are useful and effective in data with many variables.
3. They do not use prior distribution functions, and no guarantee can be given that an optimal function or subset will be found.
4. Solutions should be tested against the results from traditional analysis methods like regression models.
5. In our example of 55 patients with Marfan syndrome evolutionary operations were effective to identify a subset of genes discriminating between patients with large and small aortas at $p < 0.0001$. A standard logistic regression of the best fit genes produced a multiple correlation coefficient of 0.878, indicating that the selected genes were very good predictors of large aortas.

References

1. Akbari R, Ziarati K (2011) A multilevel evolutionary algorithm for optimizing numerical functions. Int J Ind Eng Comput 2:419–430
2. R Package Subselect (2013) www.r-statistics.com. 16 Aug 2013
3. Radonic T, de Witte P, Groenink M, de Waard V, Lutter R, van Eijk M, Jansen M, Timmermans J, Kempers M, Scholte AJ, Hilhorst-Hofstee Y, van den Berg MP, Van Tintelen

JP, Pals G, Baars MJ, Mulder BJ, Zwinderman AH (2012) Inflammation aggravates disease
severity in Marfan syndrome patients. PLoS One 7:e32963
4. Vinterbo S, Ohno L (1999) A genetic algorithm to select variables in logistic regression:
example in the domain of myocardial infarction. In: Proceedings of the AMIA (American
Medical Information Association) symposium, Washington DC, USA, pp 984–988

Chapter 3
Multiple Treatments

1 Summary

1.1 Background

Clinical studies often assess the efficacy of multiple treatments and are at risk of increased type I errors due to multiple testing.

1.2 Objective

To review methods for adjusting the type I errors.

1.3 Methods

Using a real data example we reviewed the LSD (least squares difference), HSD (Tukey's honesty significant difference), Bonferroni, and the Dunnett tests.

1.4 Results

The LSD test provided p-values of 0.01, 0.001, 0.017, 0.03, the HSD and Bonferroni tests only provided a single significant p-value at 0.005 and 0.006, the Dunnett test provided two significant tests at p = 0.035 and 0.002.

T.J. Cleophas and A.H. Zwinderman, *Machine Learning in Medicine: Part Three*,
DOI 10.1007/978-94-007-7869-6_3, © Springer Science+Business Media Dordrecht 2013

1.5   Conclusions

1. Multiple testing is very common when testing clinical data files, particularly, big computer data files, and such files are at risk of major type I errors of finding an effect where there is none.
2. Often such data files can only be analyzed using machine learning methodologies.
3. Multiple testing adjustments are scarcely included in these machine learning methodologies.
4. Investigators have to find out for themselves how to adjust multiple testing, if commands for the purpose are not available in the software.
5. LSD, HSD, Bonferroni, Dunnett methods for adjustments are explained, and were adequate in the examples given.

2   Introduction

Clinical studies often assess the efficacy of more than one new treatment. Treatments are often called exposure variables. Personal factors, like gender, age class, comorbidities are, generally, also considered as exposure variables, but they are, usually, not taken into account in randomized trials, because their effects tend to even out in the randomization process. However, in non-randomized research they have to be included in the analysis to rule out confounding and interaction.

The assessment of multiple treatments with or without additional exposure variables introduces another problem: the statistical problem of multiple testing, which increases the risk of false positive statistical results, and thus increases the type-I error risk. Multiple testing is particularly common with modern computer data files involving big data, hundreds of variables like genes and other laboratory values, and it produces easily hundreds of p-values. A p-value of 5 % means that we have the chance of a type I error (finding a difference where there is none) of 5 %. With two tests the chance of at least once 5 % is twice, and is thus 10 %. With hundreds of p-values many "so-called" significant ones are found: usually about 5 out of 100 if the p-value for significance is defined 5 %. They do not indicate true significant effects in the data, but, rather, multiple type I errors. This problem requires that the risk of the type I error is adjusted, preferably at the 5 % level.

The problem of multiple testing is particularly an issue with machine learning methodologies, like cluster analysis [1], neural networks [2], factor analysis [3], Bayesian networks [4], support vector machines [5] etc. Unlike traditional clinical trials, with a single endpoint and treatment modality, these methodologies can not be adequately analyzed with traditional prospective null hypothesis tests. Multiple testing is routine, and adjustments for it is scarcely included in these machine learning methodologies. This chapter was written as a warning to investigators that they should take care and perform post hoc assessments for themselves if commands are not given in the machine learning software. Recommendations for making choices and stepwise analyses using real data examples are included.

3 Multiple Treatments

When in a trial three of more treatments are compared to each other, the typical first statistical analysis is to test the null hypothesis (H0) of no difference between treatments versus the alternative hypothesis (H$_a$) that at least one treatment deviates from the others. Suppose that in the trial k different treatments are compared, then the null hypothesis is formulated as H0 : $\vartheta_1 = \vartheta_2 = \ldots = \vartheta_k$, where ϑ_i is the expected treatment-effect of treatment i. When the efficacy variable is quantitative (and normally distributed), then ϑ is the mean value. When the efficacy variable is binary (e.g. healthy or ill), then ϑ is the proportion of positive (say healthy) patients. When the efficacy variable is of ordinal character, or is a survival time, ϑ can have different quantifications. For the remainder of this paragraph we assume that the efficacy is quantitative and normally distributed, because for this situation the multiple testing procedure has been studied thoroughestly.

Consider the randomized clinical trial comparing five different treatments for ejaculation praecox [6]: one group of patients received a placebo treatment (group 1), and the four other groups received different serotonin reuptake inhibitors (SSRI). The primary variable for evaluating the efficacy was the logarithmically transformed intravaginal ejaculation latency time (IELT) measured after 6 weeks of treatment. The null hypothesis in this trial was that there was no difference between the five groups of patients with respect to the mean of the logarithmically transformed IELT: H0 : $\vartheta_1 = \vartheta_2 = \vartheta_3 = \vartheta_4 = \vartheta_5$. The summarized data of this trial are listed in Table 3.1.

The first statistical analysis was performed by computing an analysis of variance (ANOVA) table. The F-test for the testing the null hypothesis had value 4.13 with 4 and 39 degrees of freedom and p-value 0.0070. The within group sums of squares was 55.16 with 39 degrees of freedom, thus the mean squared error was S = 1.41. Since the p-value was far below the nominal level of $\alpha = 0.05$, the null hypothesis could be rejected. This led to the not-too-informative conclusion that not all population averages were equal. A question immediately encountered is which one of the different populations did and which one did not differ from each other.

Table 3.1 Randomized clinical trial comparing five different treatments for ejaculation praecox [6]: one group of patients received a placebo treatment (group 1), and the four other groups received different serotonin reuptake inhibitors (SSRI)

Treatment	Sample size n	Mean s	Standard deviation S
Placebo	9	3.34	1.14
SSRI A	6	3.96	1.09
SSRI B	7	4.96	1.18
SSRI C	12	5.30	1.51
SSRI D	10	4.70	0.78

The primary variable for evaluating the efficacy was the logarithmically transformed intravaginal ejaculation latency time (IELT) measured after 6 weeks of treatment

This question concerns the problem of multiple testing or post-hoc comparison of treatment groups.

The only way of finding out which one of the populations means differ from each other is to compare every treatment group with all of the other groups or with a specified subset receiving other treatments. When there are 5 different treatments, $5 \times 4/2 = 10$ different pairs of treatments can be compared. In general, when there are k treatments, k $(k-1)/2$ different comparisons can be made.

The easiest approach to this question is to calculate the Student's t-test for each comparison of the groups i and j. This procedure may be refined by using in the denominator of the t-test the pooled-within-group variance S_w^2, as already calculated in the above F-test according to:

$$t_{ij} = \frac{\overline{x}_i - \overline{x}_j}{\sqrt{S_w^2 \left(\frac{1}{n_i} + \frac{1}{n_j} \right)}}. \qquad (3.1)$$

This t-statistic has n-k degrees of freedom, where n is the total number of observations in the entire sample and k is the number of treatment groups. This procedure is called the "least significant difference" procedure (LSD procedure). For the application of the LSD procedure, it is essential to perform it sequentially to a significant F-test of the ANOVA procedure. So if one chooses to perform the LSD procedure, one first calculates the ANOVA procedure and stops if the F-test is non-significant, and calculates the LSD tests only if the F-test is statistically significant.

When the different treatment groups are compared without performing ANOVA first, or when you do so without the F-test being significant, then the problem of multiple comparisons is, particularly, enhanced. This means that when you make enough comparisons, the chance of finding a significant difference will be substantially larger than the nominal level of $\alpha = 0.05$: thus the risk of a type-I error will be (far) too large. There may be situations where we want to further the analysis all the same.

4   Explanation of the Meaning of the Type I and II Errors

H1, the hypothesis 1, (Fig. 3.1) is a graph based on the data of our trial (mean $\pm$ standard error of the mean (SEM)). H0, the hypothesis 0, is the same graph with mean 0 (mean $\pm$ SEM). H1 is also the summary of the means of many trials similar to our trial, H0 is also the summary of many trials similar to our trial but with an overall effect of 0. If hypothesis is true, then the mean of our study is part of H0, if H1 is true, then the mean of our study is part of H1. So, the mean of our study may be part of H0 or H1. We can't prove, but calculate the chance of either these two possibilities.

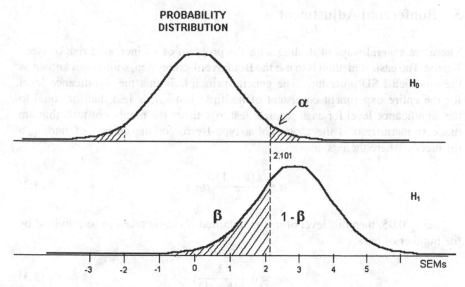

Fig. 3.1 Two Gaussian like, frequency distribution curves. H1, the hypothesis 1, is the curve based on the data of our trial (mean ± standard error of the mean (SEM)); H0, the hypothesis 0, is the same curve with mean 0 (mean ± SEM); α = type I error; β = type II error

A mean of approximately 3 SEMs is far from 2.101 (the x-axis value consistent with a p-value of 5 %. Suppose our study belongs to H0. Only 5 % of the H0 trials are >2.101 SEMs distant from 0. The chance that our study belongs to H0 is <5 %.We will reject this small possibility. Suppose our study belongs to H1. Up to approximately 30 % of the H1 trials are <2.201 SEMs distant from 0. These 30 % cannot reject the null hypothesis of no effect. Right from 2.101 SEMs we have about 70 % of the area under the curve of H1, the studies in here can do so. We conclude that if H0 is true, we have <5 % to find it, if H1 is true, 70 % chance to find it.

Alpha (here 5 %)	
	= the outlier area under the curve of H0
	= the area of rejecting the H0
	= usually 5 %
	= chance to find a difference where there is none
	= type I error.
Beta (here approximately 30 %)	
	= left part of the area under the curve of H1
	= H1 is true but H0 cannot be rejected
	= chance to find no difference where there is one
	= type II error.

The right side of the area under the curve of H1 is 100–30 = approximately 70 % gives the power of the study.

5   Bonferroni Adjustment

There are several ways of dealing with the problem of an increased risk of type-I-error. The easiest method is to use the Bonferroni-correction, sometimes known as the modified LSD procedure. The general principle is that the significance level for the entire experiment consistent of multiple tests, α, is less than or equal to the significance level for each separate test, α_C, times the number of tests that are made (remember α is the chance of a type-I-error or the chance of finding a difference where there is none):

$$\alpha \le \frac{k(k-1)}{2}\ \alpha_C \tag{3.2}$$

If $\alpha \le 0.05$, then this level of α is maintained if , α_C is taken to be , divided by the number of tests:

$$\alpha_C = \alpha\ \frac{2}{k(k-1)}. \tag{3.3}$$

When k is not too large, this method performs well.

> E.g., 3 tests
> $\alpha = 3 \times 0.05 = 0.15$
> Bonferroni $\alpha = 0.15 \times \big(2/(3 \times 2)\big) = 0.05$
>
> E.g., 6 tests
> $\alpha = 6 \times 0.05 = 0.30$
> Bonferroni $\alpha = 0.30 \times \big(2/(6 \times 5)\big) = 0.02$

If k is large (e.g., k > 5), then the Bonferroni correction is over-conservative, meaning that the nominal significance level soon will be much lower than $\alpha = 0.05$ and loss of power occurs accordingly. This can be explained: if you artificially minimize the type I error, then the type II error increases, and consequently the power is minimized (see Fig. 3.1).

6   Alternative Methods for Adjusting Multiple Testing

There are several alternative methods [7], but here we will discuss briefly three of them: (1) Tukey's honestly significant difference (HSD) method, (2) the Student-Newman-Keuls method, and (3) the method of Dunnett. Tukey's HSD method calculates the test-statistic from the above Eq. (3.1), but determines the significance level slightly differently, by considering the distribution of the largest standardized difference $|x_i - x_j|/se_{(xi - xj)}$. This distribution is somewhat more complex than that of the t-distribution or of the LSD procedure. A table of significance levels is available in all major statistical books as well as statistical software packages such as SAS and SPSS [8, 9]. The HSD procedure controls the maximum experiment wise error rate, and performs well in simulation studies, especially when sample sizes are unequal.

The Student-Newman-Keuls (SNK) procedure is a so-called multiple-stage or multiple range test. The procedure first tests the homogeneity of all k means at the nominal level α_k. When the homogeneity is rejected, then each subset of (k−1) means is tested for homogeneity at the nominal level α_{k-1}, and so on. It does so by calculating the studentized statistic in the above Eq. (3.1) for all pairs. The distribution of this statistic is again rather complex, and it depends on the degrees of freedom n-k (from ANOVA), on the number of comparisons that are made, and on α_k. The table of significance levels is likewise available in most statistical packages. The conclusions of the SNK procedure critically depend on the order of the pair wise comparisons being made. The proper procedure is to compare first the largest mean with the smallest, then the largest with the second-smallest, and so on. An important rule is that if no significant difference exists between two means, it should be concluded that no difference exists between any means enclosed by the two, without further need of testing.

There are many multiple range tests [7], mainly differing in their use of the significance level α_k, and α_{k-1}. The Student-Newman-Keuls procedure uses $\alpha_k = \alpha = 0.05$, and therefore does not control the maximum experiment-wise error rate.

Finally, there is a special multiple comparison procedure for comparing all active treatments to a control or placebo group. This is the Dunnett's procedure. For all treatments the studentized statistic of above Eq. (3.1) compared to the placebo group is calculated. In case of Dunnett's procedure, this statistic again has a complex distribution (many-one t-statistic) which depends on the number of active treatment groups, the degrees of freedom and a correlation term which depends on the sample sizes in each treatment group. Tables are likewise available in statistical packages. If sample sizes are not equal, it is important to use the harmonic mean of the sample sizes when calculating the significance of the Dunnett test.

7 Statistical Packages

Most of the statistical packages compute common multiple range tests, and provide associated confidence intervals for the difference in means. In our trial comparing 4 SSRIs and placebo in patients with ejaculation praecox, we were interested in all

Table 3.2 In the trial from Table 3.1 the investigators were interested in all of the possible comparisons between the five treatment groups

		Difference	P value			
		Mean (SE)	LSD	HSD	Bonferroni	Dunnett
Placebo vs.	A	−0.62 (0.63)	0.33	0.86	0.99	0.73
	B	−1.62 (0.60)	0.01	0.07	0.10	0.035
	C	−1.96 (0.52)	0.001	0.005	0.006	0.002
	D	−1.36 (0.55)	0.017	0.12	0.17	0.058
A vs.	B	−1.00 (0.66)	0.14	0.56	0.99	
	C	−1.34 (0.60)	0.03	0.18	0.30	
	D	−0.74 (0.61)	0.24	0.75	0.99	
B vs.	C	−0.34 (0.57)	0.56	0.98	0.99	
	D	0.26 (0.59)	0.66	0.99	0.99	
C vs.	D	0.60 (0.51)	0.25	0.76	0.99	

Since the ANOVA F-test was statistically significant, we applied the LSD procedure to find out which treatment differed significantly from each other. We found the following results. HSD procedure, the Bonferroni correction, and Dunnett's procedure of the same data were applied for control

SE = standard error

of the possible comparisons between the five treatment groups. In SPSS [9] the following commands are given:

> Command: Menu....Analyze....Compare Means....One-way Anova....Dependent List: IELT (ejaculation latency time)....Factor: Treatments....click Post Hoc Comparisons.... mark LSD, Bonferroni, Dunnett, Tukey (= HSD)....click Continue....click OK.

Since the ANOVA F-test was statistically significant, we applied the LSD procedure to find out which treatment differed significantly from each other. We found the following results. HSD procedure, the Bonferroni correction, and Dunnett's procedure of the same data were applied for control (Table 3.2).

The mean difference indicates the differences of the means of the groups as shown in Table 3.2. The standard error as calculated from the studentized statistic in the Eq. (3.1), and is required in order to construct confidence intervals. The critical values for the construction of such confidence intervals are supplied by appropriate tables for the HSD, and Dunnett's procedure, but are also calculated by most statistical software programs. In our case it is obvious that the LSD procedure provides the smallest p-values, and significant differences between SSRIs B, C and D and placebo results, as well as between A and C results. When using the Bonferroni test or the HSD procedure, only SSRI C is significantly different from placebo. Dunnett's test agrees with the LSD procedure with respect to the differences of the SSRIs compared to placebo, but has no information on the differences between the SSRIs.

8 Discussion

There is no general consensus on what post-hoc test to use or when to use it; as the statistical community has not yet reached agreement on this issue. The US Food and Drug Agency suggests in its clinical trial handbook for in house usage to describe in the study protocol the arguments for using a specific method, but refrains from making any preference. We have a light preference for calculating an overall test first such as is done with ANOVA, and subsequently proceed with the LSD test.

Unfortunately, so far multiple comparisons methods have not been developed much for discrete, ordinal and censored data. When dealing with such data, it is best to perform first an overall test by chi-square, Kruskal-Wallis or logrank methods, and afterwards perform pair wise comparisons with a Bonferroni correction.

Whatever method for multiple comparisons, its use or the lack of its use should be discussed in the statistical analysis, and preferably be specified in the analysis plan of the study protocol.

9 Conclusions

1. Multiple testing is very common when testing clinical data files, particularly, big computer data files, and such files are at risk of major type I errors of finding an effect where there is none.
2. Often, such files can only be analyzed using machine learning methodologies.
3. Multiple testing adjustments are scarcely included in these machine learning methodologies.
4. Investigators have to find out for themselves how to adjust multiple testing if commands for the purpose are not available in the software.
5. LSD, HSD, Bonferroni, Dunnett methods for adjustments are explained, and were adequate in the examples given.

References

1. Cleophas TJ, Zwinderman AH (2013) Hierarchical cluster analysis for unsupervised data. In: Cleophas TJ, Zwinderman AH (eds) Machine learning in medicine. Springer, Heidelberg, pp 183–195
2. Cleophas TJ, Zwinderman AH (2013) Artificial intelligence, multilayer perceptron modeling. In: Cleophas TJ, Zwinderman AH (eds) Machine learning in medicine. Springer, Heidelberg, pp 145–154
3. Cleophas TJ, Zwinderman AH (2013) Factor analysis. In: Cleophas TJ, Zwinderman AH (eds) Machine learning in medicine. Springer, Heidelberg, pp 167–181
4. Cleophas TJ, Zwinderman AH (2013) Bayesian networks. In: Cleophas TJ, Zwinderman AH (eds) Machine learning in medicine, part two. Springer, Heidelberg, pp 163–170
5. Cleophas TJ, Zwinderman AH (2013) Support vector machines. In: Cleophas TJ, Zwinderman AH (eds) Machine learning in medicine, part two. Springer, Heidelberg, pp 155–161

6. Waldinger MD, Hengeveld MW, Zwinderman AH, Olivier B (1998) Effect of SSRI antide-
   pressants on ejaculation: a double-blind, randomized, placebo-controlled study with fluoxetine,
   fluvoxamine, paroxetine, and sertraline. J Clin Psychopharmacol 18:274–281
7. Anonymous (1999) Multiple comparisons book. Edition University of Leiden, Leiden
8. SAS Statistical Software (2013) www.sas.com. 17 June 2013
9. SPSS Statistical Software (2013) www.spss.com. 17 June 2013

Chapter 4
Multiple Endpoints

1 Summary

1.1 Background

Multiple endpoints is a multiple testing problem and is very common when analyzing clinical data.

1.2 Objective

To review the possible solutions for this problem

1.3 Methods

Examples from the literature and from the authors' own research are given.

1.4 Results and Conclusions

1. There is no consensus within the statistical community on how to cope with multiple endpoints.
2. Particularly, composite endpoints and reducing the numbers of endpoints are the best powered solutions.
3. Bonferroni and Hochberg are not entirely adequate, because the endpoints can not be considered to be independent of one another.

T.J. Cleophas and A.H. Zwinderman, *Machine Learning in Medicine: Part Three*,
DOI 10.1007/978-94-007-7869-6_4, © Springer Science+Business Media Dordrecht 2013

4. The result of a multivariate analysis is often hard to interpret and requires post hoc tests, e.g., multiple ANOVAs (analyses of variance), that are, of course, at risk of new type I errors.
5. Multivariate tests are for most data not very powerful, and their results are, generally, pretty meaningless, if a sound hypothesis for the complex model is lacking, and the purpose is explorative.
6. Advantages of it are the following:

   (1) type I errors are reduced,
   (2) it looks at interactions between dependent variables,
   (3) it can sometimes detect subgroup properties and include them in the analysis,
   (4) it can occasionally unmask otherwise underpowered effects.

2   Introduction

Machine learning has simplified the analysis not only of multiple treatments as discussed in the previous chapter, but also the analysis of multiple endpoints. Examples of methods doing the latter are discriminant analysis [1], and partial least squares [2].

Similarly to multiple predictor data like multiple treatments, multiple endpoint data are at increased risks of type I errors of finding differences where there are none. Several ways of handling the problem here are possible. This chapter reviews six of them. Mostly, clinical efficacy studies use several, and sometimes many, endpoints to evaluate the treatment efficacy. The use of significance tests separately for each endpoint increases the risk of finding differences where there is none: e.g. if the risk of finding a difference by chance is 5 % with one endpoint, then it will be 10 % with two endpoints etc. The statistical analysis should reflect awareness of this very problem, and in the study protocol the use or non-use of statistical adjustments or their lack must be explained. There are several ways of handling this problem of multiple endpoints which is, similarly to that of multiple treatments, a problem of multiple testing.

We will use real data examples and step by step analyse for the benefit of the investigators.

3   Reducing the Numbers of Endpoints

The most obvious way is to simply reduce the number of endpoint parameters otherwise called primary outcome variable. Preferably, we should include one primary parameter, usually being the variable that provides the most relevant and convincing evidence of the primary objective of the trial. The trial success is formulated in terms of results demonstrated by this very variable, and prior sample size determination is also based on this variable. Other endpoint variables are placed on a lower level of importance and are defined secondary variables. The secondary variable results may be used to support the evidence provided by the primary variable.

It may sometimes be desirable to use two or more primary variables, each of which sufficiently important for display in the primary analysis. The statistical analysis of such an approach should be carefully spelled in the protocol. In particular, it should be stated in advance what result of any of these variables is least required for the purpose of meeting the trial objectives. Of course, if the purpose of the trial is to demonstrate a significant effect in two or more variables, then there is no need for adjustment of the type-I error risk, but the consequence is that the trial fails in its objectives if one of these variables do not produce a significant result. Obviously, such a rule enhances the chance of erroneously negative trials, in a way similar to the risk of negative trials due to small sample sizes.

4   A Pragmatic Approach

A different more philosophical approach to the problem of multiple outcome variables is to informally integrate the data and look for trends without judging one or two low P-values among otherwise high P-values as proof. This requires discipline and is particularly efficient when multiple measurements are performed for the purpose of answering one single question, e.g., the benefit to health of a new drug estimated in terms of effect on mortality in addition to a number of morbidity variables. There is nothing wrong with this practice. We should not make any formal correction for multiple comparisons of this kind. Instead, we should informally integrate all the data before reaching a conclusion. A problem is that clinical investigators and physicians frequently want hard data, not meaningless p-values.

5   Bonferroni Correction

An alternative way of dealing with the multiple comparison problem when there are many primary variables, is to apply a Bonferroni correction. This means that *the p-value of every variable is multiplied by the number of endpoints k.* This ensures that if treatments were truly equivalent, the trial as a whole will have less than a 5 % chance of getting any p-value less than 0.05; thus the overall type-I error rate will be less than 5 %.

6 Hochberg's Procedure

The Bonferroni correction, however, is not entirely correct when multiple comparisons are dependent of each other (multiple comparisons in one subject cannot be considered independent of each other, see Chap. 2, Sect. 3, for additional discussion of this issue). Also the Bonferroni correction explained in the previous chapter is an overcorrection in case of larger numbers of endpoints, particularly when different endpoints are (highly) correlated. A somewhat more adequate variation of the Bonferroni correction, was suggested by Hochberg [3]. *When there are k primary values, the idea is to multiply the largest p-value with 1, the second-largest p-value with 2, the third largest p-value with 3, . . ., and the smallest p-value with k.* We do not attempt to explain the mathematical arguments of this procedure, but conclude that lowest and highest −values will be less different from each other. In practice, Hochberg's procedure is frequently hardly less conservative than is the Bonferroni correction.

7 Composite Endpoints

A further alternative for analyzing two or more primary variables is to design a summary measure or composite variable. With such an approach endpoint and primary variables must, of course, be assessed in advance, , and the algorithm to calculate the composite must also be specified a priori. Since in this case primary variables are reduced to one composite, there is no need to make adjustments to salvage the type-I error rate. For the purpose of appropriate composite variables there are a few sensible rules to bear in mind:

Highly correlated variables, measuring more or less the same patient characteristic can best be replaced with their average. In this way the number of primary variables is reduced, and an additional advantage is that the mean is more reliable than single measurements.

When the variables have different scales (e.g. blood pressure is measured in mm Hg units, and cholesterol in mmol/L units), the composite variables are best calculated as standardized variables. This means that the overall mean is subtracted from each measurement and that the resulting difference is divided by the overall standard deviation. In this way all variables will have zero mean and unit standard deviation in the total sample.

Well-known examples of composite variables are rating scales routinely used for the assessment of health-related quality of life, as well as disease-activity-scales (e.g., the disease activity scale of Fuchs for patients with rheumatoid arthritis,

Table 4.1 Clinical trial of patients with atherosclerosis comparing 2-year placebo versus pravastatin medication [6]

Change of:	Placebo (n = 31)	Pravastatin (n = 48)	P^a	P^b	P^c
Total cholesterol decrease	−0.07 (0.72)	0.25 (0.73)	0.06	0.24	0.11
HDL cholesterol increase	−0.02 (0.18)	0.04 (0.12)	0.07	0.28	0.11
LDL cholesterol decrease	0.34 (0.60)	0.59 (0.65)	0.09	0.36	0.11
Triglycerides increase	0.03 (0.65)	0.28 (0.68)	0.11	0.44	0.11

The efficacy of this medication was evaluated by assessing the change of total cholesterol, HDL cholesterol, LDL cholesterol, and triglycerides. The mean changes and standard deviations (mmol/L) are given, while also the uncorrected p-values, and the corrected p-values according to Bonferroni and Hochberg are reported
[a]p-value of Student's t-test
[b]Bonferroni corrected p-value
[c]p-value corrected using Hochberg's methods

DAS [4]). The DAS is a composite based on the Ritchie joint pain score, the number of swollen joints, and, in addition, the erythrocyte sedimentation rate:

$$DAS = 0.53938\sqrt{ritchie\ index} + 0.06465\,(number\ of\ swollen\ joints)$$
$$+ 0.330\ln(erythocyte\ sedimentation\ rate) + 0.224.$$

For the statistical analysis of a composite variable, standard methods may be used without adjustments. Lauter [5] showed that the statistical test for the composite has 5 % type-I error rate. He also showed that such a statistical test is especially sensitive when each endpoint variable has more or less the same individual p-value, but that it has little sensitivity when one endpoint variable is much more significant than others.

We applied these methods to a clinical trial of patients with atherosclerosis comparing 2-year placebo versus pravastatin medication [6]. The efficacy of this medication was evaluated by assessing the change of total cholesterol, HDL cholesterol, LDL cholesterol, and triglycerides. The mean changes and standard deviations (mmol/L) are given in Table 4.1, while also the uncorrected p-values, and the corrected p-values according to Bonferroni and Hochberg are reported.

It is obvious that none of the changes are statistically significant using a standard t-test, but it is also clear that all four efficacy variables have a treatment difference that points in the same direction, namely of a positive pravastatin effect. When correcting for multiple testing, the p-values are nowhere near statistical significance. A composite variable of the form z = (total cholesterol + HDL + LDL + triglycerides)/4, where the four lipid measurements are standardized, however, did show statistically significant results: the mean of Z in the placebo group was −0.23 (SD 0.59), and the mean of Z in the pravastatin group was 0.15 (SD 0.56), different $p < 0.01$, and so, it is appropriate to conclude that pravastatin significantly reduced the composite variable.

8   Multivariate Analysis

Finally, there are several multivariate methods to perform an overall statistical test for which the type-I error risk equals 5 %. Equivalently to the situation comparing many different treatment groups, one might argue that the overall test controls the type-I error, and that subsequently to the overall test, one can perform t-tests and the like without adjustment to explore which variables show significant differences. For comparing two treatment groups on several (normally distributed) variables, one may use Hotelling's T-square, which is the multivariate generalization of the Student's t-test. Other methods to compare different groups of patients on several variables are discriminant analysis, variants of principal components analysis and multinomial logistic regression. The discussion of these methods falls outside the scope of this chapter, but will be addressed in more detail in the Chaps. 21 and 25. It suffices to remark that Hotelling's T-square [7] and the other multivariate methods are readily available through most statistical packages. E.g., in SPSS [8] the commands are given.

> Command: Menu....Analyze....General Linear Model .... Multivariate ....Dependent variables: enter the y-variables, the endpoints (continuous variables)....Fixed factor: enter the x-variable, a binary variable.... Options....Display: mark Descriptives....mark Homogeneity tests....click Continue....click OK.

A table with four multivariate tests are given: Pillai's, Wilk's Lambda, Hotelling's Trace, and Roy's Largest Root. All of the tests generally are based on normal distributions and homogeneity of variables, and are, approximately, equally robust.

9   Discussion

Multiple endpoints is a very common problem when analyzing clinical trials. There is no consensus within the statistical community on how to cope with these problems. It is, therefore, essential, that awareness of the existence of these problems is reflected in the study protocol and the statistical analysis. A series of solutions are given. Particularly, composite endpoint and reducing the number of endpoints are the best powered solutions. Bonferroni and Hochberg are not entirely adequate, because the endpoints can not be considered to be independent of one another. The result of a multivariate analysis is often hard to interpret and requires post hoc tests, e.g., multiple ANOVAs (analyses of variance), that are of course at risk of new type I errors. Multivariate tests are for most data not very powerful, and their results are, generally, pretty meaningless, particularly, if a sound hypothesis for the complex model is lacking, and the purpose is explorative. Advantages of it are the following.

1. The risks of type I errors are reduced.
2. It looks at interactions between dependent variables.
3. It can sometimes detect subgroup properties and include them in the analysis,
4. It can occasionally unmask otherwise underpowered effects.

10 Conclusions

1. Multiple endpoints is a multiple testing problem and is very common when analyzing clinical trials.
2. There is no consensus within the statistical community on how to cope with it.
3. Particularly, composite endpoint and reducing the number of endpoints are the best powered solutions.
4. Bonferroni and Hochberg are not entirely adequate, because the endpoints can not be considered to be independent of one another.
5. The result of a multivariate analysis is often hard to interpret and requires post hoc tests, e.g., multiple ANOVAs (analyses of variance), that are, of course, at risk of new type I errors.
6. Multivariate tests are for the most part not very powerful, and their (weak) results are, generally, pretty meaningless, particularly, if a sound hypothesis for the complex model is lacking, and the analysis is explorative.
7. Advantages of multivariate tests are the following:

   (1) the risks of type I errors are reduced,
   (2) it looks at interactions between dependent variables,
   (3) it can sometimes detect subgroup properties, and include them in the analysis,
   (4) it can occasionally unmask otherwise underpowered effects.

References

1. Cleophas TJ, Zwinderman AH (2012) Discriminant analysis. In: Cleophas TJ, Zwinderman AH (eds) Machine learning in medicine part one. Springer, Heidelberg, pp 215–224
2. Cleophas TJ, Zwinderman AH (2012) Partial least squares. In: Cleophas TJ, Zwinderman AH (eds) Machine learning in medicine part one. Springer, Heidelberg, pp 197–212
3. Hochberg Y (1988) A sharper Bonferroni procedure for multiple tests of significance. Biometrika 75:800–802
4. Fuchs HA (1993) The use of the disease activity score in the analysis of clinical trials in rheumatoid arthritis. J Rheumatol 20:1863–1866
5. Lauter J (1996) Exact t and F-tests for analyzing studies with multiple endpoints. Biometrics 52:964–970

6. Jukema JW, Bruschke AV, Van Boven AJ, Zwinderman AH et al (1995) Effects of lipid lowering by pravastatin on the regression of coronary artery disease in symptomatic men. Circulation 91:2528–2540
7. Cleophas TJ, Zwinderman AH (2012) Canonical regression. In: Cleophas TJ, Zwinderman AH (eds) Machine in medicine part one. Springer, Heidelberg, pp 225–240
8. SPSS Statistical Software (2013) www.spss.com. 7 Aug 2013

Chapter 5
Optimal Binning

1 Summary

1.1 Background

Optimal binning is a method for multi-interval discretization of continuous variables. It is used for classification learning, and is already widely applied in econo-/sociometrics.

1.2 Objective

To assess its efficiency in a medical research example.

1.3 Methods

A 1,445 case hypothesized example of the effects of unhealthy food/lifestyle on children's overweight.

1.4 Results

All of the 4 predictor variables were categorized into 2 or 3 bins with very different proportions of risks of children's overweights between the bins: 29.8 vs. 9.6, 20.4 vs. 43.8, 32.0 vs. 19.6, and 1.4 vs. 40.1 and 63.3 %. Model entropies, used as measures for the loss of information by the procedures, were adequately low.

T.J. Cleophas and A.H. Zwinderman, *Machine Learning in Medicine: Part Three*,   37
DOI 10.1007/978-94-007-7869-6_5, © Springer Science+Business Media Dordrecht 2013

1.5   Conclusions

1. The results of the optimal binning variables instead of the original continuous variables may either produce (1) better or (2) worse statistics, (1) better, because unnecessary noise due to the continuous scaling may be deleted, (2) worse, because information may be lost if you replace a continuous variable with a binary one.
2. Optimal binning procedure produces a type of information different from that of traditional procedures. E.g., Logistic regression of bin variables against outcome tells what happens if you go from a low to high risk bin, while traditional analysis tells what happens per unit of the predictor variable.
3. Advantages of optimal binning include:

   (1) it is more adequate than traditional regression with non-linear relationships between outcome and predictor,
   (2) it is more adequate if categories as considered are clinically more relevant,
   (3) if the original continuous variables are full of noise,
   (4) and if a binning syntax is produced which can, subsequently, be applied to future data.

4. Optimal binning can be, adequately, used for classification learning of health parameters.

2   Introduction

Optimal binning is a method for multi-interval discretization of continuous-value variables for classification learning. Continuous features are converted to discretized or nominal variables for the purpose of optimal data fitting. It was invented by Usama Fayyad, computer scientist and vice-president of Yahoo Inc, Sunnyvale, CA, USA in 1993 [1]. It is adequate for (1) modeling non-linear relationships between continuous predictor and outcome variables, (2) reporting scaled values in the form of classes, (3) density estimates of load parameters, and it is currently a widely applied form of supervised learning within the field of machine learning and computer science. Recently, it has become available in SPSS [2] and other major statistical software programs (in SPSS since November 2006, version 15.0). Though widely used in marketing research and econo-/sociometrics, it is little used in clinical research, but this is probably a matter of time. It was recently, e.g., recommended for the analysis of prognostic and health management parameters [3], and has been applied by a group of pediatricians for health education evaluation in children [4]. The current paper, using a hypothetical example of the effect of various predictors of the consumption of unhealthy food in children, was written to explain this novel method to clinical investigators. For their benefit step by step analyses are given. SPSS statistical software was used.

3 Some Theory

Optimal binning makes use of the minimum description length (MDL) methodology, a methodology based on William Ockham (1347)'s razor. The term razor is a metaphor of the "lex parsimoniae" (latin), which tells, that, among competing hypotheses, the one with the fewest assumptions should be preferred. This theory is an important concept not only in learning theory, but also in current information technology. A numerical example is given.

x =	1.0	y =	3.0
	1.3		3.3
	2.4		4.4
	3.6		5.6
	4.7		6.7

The above ten values can be described in a less lengthy way, namely

x =	1.0
	1.3
	2.4
	3.6
	4.7

and

$$y = x + 2$$

The above summary of the ten values only requires 6 instead of 10 formulations, and is, thus, considerably shorter, and, thus, more efficient to describe these data. For other data sets other models may be more efficient. MDL technology looks for any regularity in the data that can be used to compress the data, like the regularity "+2" in the above example. The most drastic data reduction is currently obtained by use of the optimal binning technique. Using iterations the computer is capable to reduce data sets of many thousands of values to just a few categories with characteristics important to the investigators. As an example, in a data set of 1,445 families the consumption of fruit/vegetable per week is assessed. We wish to categorize the data into the best fit two categories (bins) with large or low consumptions.

The iteration program of the optimal binning software, making use of the presence or absence of overweight children in the families as supervisor variable (yes or no), calculated that a minimum description length of two bins was obtained with the following results:

Bin 1: 1,142 families score over 14 units of fruit/vegetable per week for their children
Bin 2: 303 families score less than 14 units per week for their children.
Bin 1: the proportion overweight children = 340/1,142 = 0.298 ≈ 30 %
Bin 2: the proportion overweight children = 29/303 = 0.096 ≈ 10 %.

There is a large difference in proportion of overweight children in the two bins and the two bins can be used as a variable for making prediction about overweight children instead of the separate overweight value of the 1,445 families.

The optimal binning program also assesses the goodness of the binning procedure making use of the model entropy, to be interpreted as the information loss by a specific binning procedure. Model entropy, thus, estimates the usefulness of the bin model as predictor model, here, for probability of overweight: the smaller the entropy, the better the model. The worst possible entropy is no better than guessing, and is calculated as the overall entropy of the dataset, in our example, according to:

(families with overweight children)/(all families included)	$= 369/1445,$
$369/1{,}445$	$= 0.2554,$
worst entropy	$= -0.2554 \times {}^2\log (0.2554) -$
	$\quad 0.7446 \times {}^2\log (0.7446),$
${}^2\log (0.2554)$	$= \log (0.2554)/\log 2,$
worst entropy	$= 0.5029 + 0.3168 = 0.8197.$

The entropies as observed in the analysis are somewhat better, and are between 0.790 and 0.805, suggesting that the optimal binning procedure produced bin variables that may make a better prediction than that of the un-binned data set.

4 Example

A hypothesized example was used. One of the parents of 1,445 families were questioned about the presence of overweight children, the food consumption patterns of their children including the fruit/vegetable, the fastfood meal, and the unhealthy snack consumption, and the physical activities scores. SPSS was used for data analysis. The data file entitled "chap5optimalbinning.sav" can be downloaded from the internet at extras.springer.com.

Command: Transform….Optimal Binning….Variables into Bins: enter fruit/vegetables, unhealthysnacks, fastfoodmeal, physicalactivities….

Optimize Bins with Respect to: enter "overweightchildren"….click Output….Display: mark Endpoints….mark Descriptive statistics….mark Model Entropy….click Save: mark Create variables that contain binned data….Save Binning Rules as Syntax: File: enter binningchildren'shealth ….click browse and select map in your computer and save for later ….click OK.

In the output tables the Table 5.1 is given. N = the number of adults in the analysis, Minimum/Maximum = the range of the original continuous variables, Number of Distinct Values = the separate values of the continuous variables as used in the binning process, Number of Bins = the number of bins (= categories) generated and is smaller than the initials separate values of the same variables. Model Entropy (Table 5.2) gives estimates of the usefulness of the bin models as

Table 5.1 N = number of adults in the analysis, Minimum/Maximum gives the range of the original continuous variables, Number of Distinct Values = the separate values of the continuous variables as used in the binning process, Number of Bins = the number bins (= categories) generated and is smaller than the initials separate values of the same variables

Descriptive statistics

	N	Minimum	Maximum	Number of distinct values	Number of bins
fruitvegetables/wk	1,445	0	34	33	2
unhealthysnacks/wk	1,445	0	42	1,050	3
fastfoodmeal/wk	1,445	0	21	1,445	2
physicalactivities/wk	1,445	0	10	1,385	2

Table 5.2 Model Entropy gives estimates of the usefulness of the bin models as predictor models for probability of overweight: the smaller the entropy, the better the model

Model entropy

	Model entropy
fruitvegetables/wk	,790
unhealthysnacks/wk	,720
fastfoodmeal/wk	,786
physicalactivities/wk	,805

The entropies observed in the analysis are somewhat better, and vary from 0.790 to 0.805 suggesting that the optimal binning procedure produces variables that may make better predictions than those from the entire data set

Smaller model entropy indicates higher predictive accuracy of the binned variable on guide variable overweight children

predictor models for probability of overweight: the smaller the entropy, the better the model. E.g., the summary of fruitvegetables/wk shows that 1,142 adults, all scoring over 14 units of fruit/vegetable per week, are put into bin 1 and 303, all scoring less than 14 units per week, are put into bin 2 (Table 5.3).

The proportion of overweight children is much larger in bin 1 than it is in bin 2:

$$340/1,142 = 0.298 \text{ and}$$
$$29/303 = 0.096.$$

The worst possible entropy is no better than guessing. It can be calculated for the dataset according to:

$$(\text{adults with overweight children})/(\text{all adults included}) = 369/1,445 = 0.2554$$

$$\text{Worst entropy} = -0.2554 \times {}^2\log(0.2554) - 0.7446 \times {}^2\log(0.7446)$$
$${}^2\log(0.2554) = \log(0.2554)/\log 2$$
$$\text{Worst entropy} = 0.5029 + 0.3168 = 0.8197.$$

Table 5.3 The summary of fruitvegetables/wk shows that 1,142 adults, all scoring under 14 units of fruit/vegetable per week, are put into bin 1 and 303, all scoring over 14 units per week, are put into bin 2

fruitvegetables/wk

	End point		Number of cases by level of overweight children		
Bin	Lower	Upper	No	Yes	Total
1	a	14	802	340	1,142
2	14	a	274	29	303
Total			1,076	369	1,445

The proportion of overweight children is much larger in bin 1 than it is in bin 2:
$$340/1{,}142 = 0.298 \text{ and}$$
$$29/303 = 0.096$$
Each bin is computed as Lower <=fruitvegetables/wk < Upper
[a]Unbounded

Table 5.4 The summary of fastfoodmeal/wk shows that 1,125 adults, all scoring under 2 units per week, are put into bin 1 and 320, all scoring over 2 units or less per week, are put into bin 2

fastfoodmeal/wk

	End point		Number of cases by level of overweight children		
Bin	Lower	Upper	No	Yes	Total
1	a	2	896	229	1,125
2	2	a	180	140	320
Total			1,076	369	1,445

The proportion of overweight children is much larger in bin 2 than it is in bin 1:
$$229/1{,}125 = 0.204 \text{ and}$$
$$140/320 = 0.438$$
Each bin is computed as Lower < =fastfoodmeal/wk < Upper.
[a]Unbounded

The entropies observed in the analysis are somewhat better, and vary from 0.790 to 0.805 suggesting that the optimal binning procedure produces variables that may make better predictions than those from the entire data set.

The Tables 5.3, 5.4, 5.5, and 5.6 give the structure of the bins for all of the four unhealthy food/physical activities variables. All of the bins show major differences in proportions of overweight children. Table 5.6 shows that the unhealthy snack variable is binned into three rather than two categories.

When we return to the dataview pages of the software program, we will observe that the four variables have been added in the form of bin variables (with suffix_bin). They can, e.g., be used as outcome variables for making predictions about other variables like personal characteristics of parents. When turning to the

Table 5.5 The summary of physicalactivities/wk shows that 690 adults, all scoring under 8 units per week, are put into bin 1 and 755, all scoring over 8 units or less per week, are put into bin 2

physicalactivities/wk

Bin	End point		Number of cases by level of overweight children		
	Lower	Upper	No	Yes	Total
1	[a]	8	469	221	690
2	8	[a]	607	148	755
Total			1,076	369	1,445

The proportion of overweight children is much larger in bin 1 than it is in bin 2:

$$221/690 = 0.320 \text{ and}$$
$$148/755 = 0.196$$

Each bin is computed as Lower $<=$ physicalactivites/week $<$ Upper
[a]Unbounded

Table 5.6 The underneath table shows the situation where the program has produced 3 instead of 2 bins. The summary of unhealthy snacks/wk shows that 973 adults, all scoring under 12 units per week, are put into bin 1 and 314, all scoring between 12 and 19 units per week, are put into bin 2, and 158 scoring over 19 units per week are put into bin 3

unhealthysnacks/wk

Bin	End point		Number of cases by level of overweight children		
	Lower	Upper	No	Yes	Total
1	[a]	12	830	143	973
2	12	19	188	126	314
3	19	[a]	58	100	158
Total			1,976	369	1,445

The proportion of overweight children are:

$$143/973 = 0.147$$
$$126/314 = 0.401$$
$$100/158 = 0.633$$

The proportion of overweight children is much larger in the bin 3 than 2, and much larger in bin 2 than in bin 1

Each bin is computed as Lower $<=$ unhealthysnacks/wk $<$ Upper
[a]Unbounded

map selected for the syntax-file, we will observe the file which cannot be opened, but can be used in optimal binnings of future data as decision rules, using the browse command again. The syntax file is given for convenience of the readers. It is entitled "chap5binningchildren'shealth.sps", and can be downloaded from the internet at extras.springer.com.

5 Discussion

Optimal binning of continuous data may be more or less sensitive than traditional continuous data analysis. On one hand noise in the data may be removed, on the other hand meaningful information may be lost. Also the optimal binning procedure produces a type of information different from that of traditional procedures. Logistic regression with children's overweights as outcome and fruit/vegetables variable as predictor is given in the Table 5.7. The odds ratios were 0.92 and 0.25, meaning that the risk of overweight 0.92 smaller per unit of fruit/week, and 0.25 smaller per bin, that is if you go from a low fruit to a high fruit bin. Similar results are observed in the Tables 5.8, 5.9, and 5.10. From these tables it can be concluded: much fruit and vegetables is particularly in the bin with few overweights, much fastfood is in the bin with much overweight, much physical activity is in the bin with little overweight, many unhealthy snacks is in the bins with much overweight. Which information is most relevant, depends on the investigators' priorities.

Advantages of optimal binning include: (1) it is more adequate than traditional regression with non-linear relationships between outcome and predictor, (2) it is more adequate if categories are requested and considered clinically more relevant, (3) if the continuous variables are full of noise. Also an advantage is that an optimal binning syntax is produced which can subsequently be applied to future data, a procedure also applied in other machine learning techniques, like cluster analysis, neural networks, vector machine, and Bayesian networks.

Table 5.7 Logistic regression with overweight children as outcome and fruit/vegetables variable as predictor

Variables in the equation							
		B	S.E.	Wald	df	Sig.	Exp(B)
Step 1[a]	fruitvegetables	−,081	,010	61,841	1	,000	,922
	Constant	−,531	,085	38,597	1	,000	,588
[a]Variable(s) entered on step 1:fruitvegetables							
Variables in the equation							
		B	S.E.	Wald	df	Sig.	Exp(B)
Step 1[a]	fruitvegetables	−1,388	,206	45,501	1	,000	,250
	Constant	,530	,234	5,108	1	,024	1,698
[a]Variable(s) entered on step 1:fruitvegetables_bin							

The odds ratios were 0.92 and 0.25, meaning that the risk of overweight 0.92 smaller per unit of fruit/week, and 0.25 smaller per bin, that is if you go from a low fruit to a high fruit bin

Table 5.8 Logistic regression with overweight children as outcome and the unhealthy snacks variable as predictor

Variables in the equation

		B	S.E.	Wald	df	Sig.	Exp(B)
Step 1[a]	Unhealthysnacks	,130	,010	169,616	1	,000	1,139
	Constant	−2,542	,137	346,627	1	,000	,079
[a]Variable(s) entered on step 1: unhealthysnacks							

Variables in the equation

		B	S.E.	Wald	df	Sig.	Exp(B)
Step 1[a]	Unhealthysnacks_bin	1,197	,089	180,591	1	,000	3,310
	Constant	−2,918	,158	340,793	1	,000	,054
[a]Variable(s) entered on step 1: unhealthysnacks_bin							

The odds ratios were 1.14 and 3.31, meaning that the risk of overweight 1.14 times larger per unhealthy snack/week, and 3.31 times larger per bin, that is if you go from a low unhealthy snack to a high unhealthy snack bin

Table 5.9 Logistic regression with overweight children as outcome and the fastfood meals variable as predictor

Variables in the equation

		B	S.E.	Wald	df	Sig.	Exp(B)
Step 1[a]	fastfoodmeal	,239	,031	60,463	1	,000	1,271
	Constant	−1,478	,082	328,423	1	,000	,288
[a]Variable(s) entered on step 1: fastfoodmeal							

Variables in the equation

		B	S.E.	Wald	df	Sig.	Exp(B)
Step 1[b]	fastfoodmeal_bin	1,113	,135	68,122	1	,000	3,043
	Constant	−2,477	,186	177,192	1	,000	,084
[a]Variable(s) entered on step 1: fastfoodmeal_bin							

The odds ratios were 1.27 and 3.04, meaning that the risk of overweight 1.27 times larger per fast food meal/week, and 3.04 times larger per bin, that is if you go from a low fastfood bin to a high fast food bin

Table 5.10 Logistic regression with overweight children as outcome and the physical activities variable as predictor

Variables in the equation

		B	S.E.	Wald	df	Sig.	Exp(B)
Step 1[a]	physicalactivities	−,101	,022	21,135	1	,000	,904
	Constant	−,362	,163	4,949	1	,026	,696
[a]Variable(s) entered on step 1: physicalactivities							

Variables in the equation

		B	S.E.	Wald	df	Sig.	Exp(B)
Step 1[a]	physicalactivities_bin	−,659	,123	28,823	1	,000	,517
	Constant	−,094	,187	,250	1	,617	,911
[a]Variable(s) entered on step 1: physicalactivities_bin							

The odds ratios were 0.90 and 0.52, meaning that the risk of overweight 0.90 times smaller per physical activity/week, and 0.512 times smaller per bin, that is if you go from a low physical activity bin to a high physical activity bin

6 Conclusions

1. The results of the optimal binning variables instead of the original continuous variables may either produce (1) better or (2) worse statistics, (1) better, because unnecessary noise due to the continuous scaling may be deleted, (2) worse, because information may be lost if your replace a continuous variable with a binary one.
2. Optimal binning procedure produces a type of information different from that of traditional procedures. E.g., Logistic regression of bin variables against outcome tells what happen if you go from a low to high risk bin while traditional analysis tells what happens per unit of the predictor variable.
3. Advantages of optimal binning include: (1) it is more adequate than traditional regression with non-linear relationships between outcome and predictor, (2) it is more adequate if categories are considered clinically more relevant, (3) and if the original continuous variables are full of noise, (4) a binning syntax is produced which can subsequently be applied to future data.

References

1. Fayyad U, Irani K (1993) Multi-interval discretization of continuous value attributes for classification learning. In: 13th International joint conference of machine learning, Los Altos
2. SPSS Statistical Software (2013) www.spss.com. 5 June 2013
3. Vichare NM, Rodgers P, Pecht MG (2013) Methods for binning and density estimates of load parameters for prognostics and health management. www.prognodics.umd.edu. 5 June 2013
4. Sepulveda MJ, Lu C, Sill S, Young J, Edington D (2010) An observational study of an employer intervention for children's healthy weight behaviors. Pediatrics 126:e1153–e1160

Chapter 6
Exact P-Values and Their Interpretation

1 Summary

1.1 Background

In marketing and business research the 5 % cut-off p-value has been largely abandoned, and replaced with exact p-values used as criterion for making decisions on the risk men are willing to take.

1.2 Objective

To assess whether in medical research the use of exact instead of cut-off p-values would be a valuable activity too.

1.3 Methods

We review the subject, both from a theoretical and practical point of view, and use real data for the purpose.

1.4 Results of Review and Conclusions

1. A p-value <0.05 gives a conditional probability: the nullhypothesis H0 can be rejected on the limitations/assumptions that

T.J. Cleophas and A.H. Zwinderman, *Machine Learning in Medicine: Part Three*,
DOI 10.1007/978-94-007-7869-6_6, © Springer Science+Business Media Dordrecht 2013

   (1) we have up to 5 % chance of a type I error of finding a difference where there
        is none,
   (2) we have 50 % chance of a type II error of finding no difference where there
        is one,
   (3) the data are normally distributed,
   (4) they follow exactly the same distribution as that of the population from
        which the sample was taken.

2. A common misunderstanding is the concept that the p-value is, actually, the
   chance that H0 is true, and, consequently that a $p > 0.05$ indicates a significant
   similarity in the data. $P > 0.05$ may, indeed, indicate similarity. However, also a
   study-sample too small or study design inadequate to detect the difference must
   be considered.
3. An advantage of the exact p-values is the possibility of more refined conclusions
   from the research: instead of concluding significantly yes/no, we are able to
   consider levels of probabilities from very likely to be true, to very likely to be
   untrue.
4. $P > 0.95$ suggests that the observed data are closer to expectation than compatible with a Gaussian frequency distribution, and such results must, therefore, be
   scrutinized.
5. A $p < 0.0001$, if power was set at 80 %, does not completely confirm the prior
   expectations of the power assessment. Therefore, such results must be scrutinized.
6. The p-values tell us the chance of making a type I error of finding a difference
   where there is none. In the 1970s exact p-values were laborious to calculate, and
   they were, generally, approximated from statistical tables, in the form of
   $p < 0.01$ or $0.05 < p < 0.10$ etc. In the past decades with the advent of computers it became easy to calculate exact p-values such as 0.840 or 0.007. The
   cut-off p-values have not been completely abandoned, but broader attention is
   given to the interpretation of the exact p-values.

2 Introduction

Clinical research is generally involved in hypotheses like "a new treatment is
efficacious, it is safe", and testing the chance that such hypotheses are true or
untrue. The nullhypothesis (H0) is used as a term to indicate that the new treatment
is not efficacious/not safe. The famous p-value is often interpreted as the probability
that the nullhypothesis is true. However, this is an overstatement. The point is that
biological processes are full of variations. Statistical tests can not give you certainties, only chances (otherwise called probabilities or likelihoods). What chances?
The chances that your hypotheses are true/untrue. What hypotheses? Many hypotheses are possible, but investigators, generally, confine themselves to the
nullhypothesis (H0, no effect in the data), and the alternative hypothesis (H1, a
real effect in the data). The true meaning of the p-value is the probability to find the
observed study result, if the H0 were true.

A more realistic interpretation of a p-value of, e.g., 5 % for the purpose of making a prediction from your study result would be:

The probability of no effect in your data is 5 % on the provision that

1. H0 is untrue,
2. H1 is true and normally distributed,
3. the data are representative of the target population (meaning the population we want to make predictions about),
4. the data have the same frequency distribution of those of the target population.

The current chapter assesses the sense and nonsense of p-values in the predictive research. The text is largely theoretical, but various real data examples are given to explain and underscore the theory.

3 Renewed Attention to the Interpretation of P-Values

The p-values tell us the chance of making a type I error of finding a difference where there is none. Generally, a cut-off p-value of 0.05 is used to reject the null-hypothesis (H0) of no difference. In the 1970s exact p-values were laborious to calculate, and they were, generally, approximated from statistical tables, in the form of $p < 0.01$ or $0.05 < p < 0.10$ etc. In the past decades with the advent of computers the job became easy [1–4]. Exact p-values such as 0.840 or 0.007 can now be obtained fast and accurately. If you enter the term p-value calculator in Google, many of them are readily available and provide you with p-values of six digits or more [5–7].

This development has lead to a renewed attention to the interpretation of p-values. In business statistics [8, 9], the 5 % cut-off p-value has been largely abandoned and replaced with exact p-values used for making decisions on the risk business men are willing to take, mostly in terms of time and costs involved. In medicine, the cut-off p-values have not been completely abandoned, but broader attention is given to the interpretation of the exact p-values, and rightly so, because they can tell us a number of relevant things in addition to the chance of making type I errors. In the current chapter standard and renewed interpretations of p-values are reviewed as far as relevant to the interpretation of clinical trials and evidence-based medicine.

4 The P-Values and Nullhypothesis Testing

Statistics gives no certainties, only chances. What chances? Chances that hypotheses are true/untrue (we accept 95 % truths). What hypotheses? E.g., no difference from a 0 effect, a real difference from a 0 effect, worse than a 0 effect. Statistics is about estimating such chances/testing such hypotheses. Trials often calculate differences

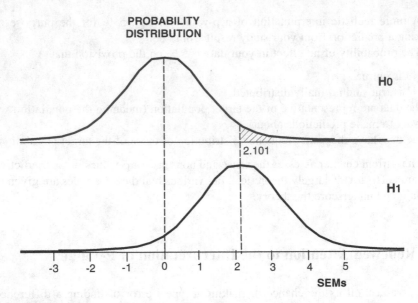

Fig. 6.1 Null-hypothesis and alternative hypothesis of a parallel group study of two groups n = 10 (18 degrees of freedom)

between test treatment and control (for example, standard treatment, placebo, baseline), and, subsequently, test whether the difference-between-the-two is different from 0.

Important hypotheses are Hypothesis 0 (H0, i.e., no difference from a 0 effect), and Hypothesis 1 (H1, the alternative hypothesis, i.e., a real difference from a 0 effect). What do these two hypotheses look like in graph? Figure 6.1 gives an example.

- H1 = graph based on the data of our trial (mean ± standard error (SEM) = 2.1 ± 1).
- H0 = same graph with mean 0 (mean ± SEM = 0 ± 1).
- Now we make a giant leap from our data to the population from which the sample was taken (we can do so, because our data are supposed to be representative of the population).

H1 =   also summary of means of many trials similar to ours (if we repeated trial, difference would be small, and distribution of means of many such trials would look like H1).

H0 =   summary of means of many trials similar to ours, but with overall effect 0 (our mean is not 0 but 2.1). Still, it could be an outlier of many studies with an overall effect of 0.

So, we should think of H0 and H1 as summaries of means of many trials.
If hypothesis 0 is true, then mean of our study is part of H0.
If hypothesis 1 is true, then mean of our study is part of H1.

We can't prove anything, but we can calculate the chance of either of these possibilities.

A mean result of 2.1 is far distant from 0:

Suppose it belongs to H0.

Only 5 % of the H0 trials >2.1 SEM distant from 0.

The chance that it belongs to H0 is <5 %.

We reject this possibility if probability is <5 %.

Suppose it belongs to H1.

50 % of the H1 trials >2.1 SEM distant from 0. These 50 % cannot reject null hypothesis, only the remainder, here also 50 %, can do so.

Conclude here if H0 is true, we have <5 % chance to find it, if H1 is true, we have 50 % chance to find it. Or in statistical terms: we reject null hypothesis of no effect at $p < 0.05$ and with a statistical power of 50 %.

Obviously, a p-value of <0.05 does not indicate a true effect, and allows for very limited conclusions [10, 11]:

1. <5 % chance to find this result if H0 is true (H0 is probably untrue, and so, this statement does not mean too much anyway);
2. only 50 % chance to find this result if H1 is true.

The conclusions illustrate the uncertainties involved in H0 – testing. With lower p-values, better certainty is provided, e.g., with $p < 0.01$ we have around 80 % chance to find this result if H1 were true, with $p < 0.001$ even 90 %. However, even then, the chance of a type II error of finding no difference where there is one is still 10 %. Also, we must realize that the above conclusions are appropriate only if

3. the data follow a normal distribution, and
4. they follow exactly the same distribution as that of the population from which the sample was taken.

5 Misunderstandings of the P-Values

The most common misunderstanding while interpreting the p-values is the concept that the p-value is actually the chance that the H0 is true, and, consequently, that $p > 0.05$ means H0 is true. Often, this result, expressed as "not significantly different from zero", is then reported as documented proof that the treatment had no effect. The distinction between demonstrating that a treatment had no effect and failing to demonstrate that it did have an effect, is subtle but very important, because the latter may be due to inadequate study methods or lack of power rather than lack of effect. Moreover, in order to assess whether the H0 is true, null-hypothesis testing can never give the answer, because this is not the issue. The only issue here is: H0 is rejected or not, no matter if it is true or untrue. To answer the question whether no-difference-in-the-data is true, we need to follow a different approach: similarity testing. With similarity (otherwise called equivalence)-testing the typical answer is: similarity is or is not demonstrated, which can be taken synonymous for no-difference-in-the-data being true or not.

6   The Determinants of the P-Values

1. *The sample size of a study*
   The t-test is helpful to understand the p-values. The p-value is equal to the area under the curve of the Gaussian-like curves of the t-tests. The values are summarized in the t-table (Table 6.1). The upper row (here called Q-values) gives the p-values associated with their t-values. The larger the degrees of freedom (left column, it corresponds to the sample size of a study), the smaller the t-values and the larger the p-values.
2. *The magnitude of the effect of a study*
   The t-table also shows that the larger the t-value, the smaller the p-value. As t = d/SE, where d = magnitude study effect and SE is its standard error, it follows that a large study effect causes a p-value to be small.
3. *The spread in the data*
   The larger the t-value, the smaller the p-value. As t = d/SE, where d = magnitude study effect and SE is its standard error (the measure of spread in the data), it follows that a large spread in the data causes a p-value to be small.

The t-values are only used in the t-test, and other tests use other test statistics, like chi-square values, F-values, z-values etc. However, the determinants of the p-values obtained from them are, largely, similar, and we can, thus, come to some relevant conclusions. It is tricky to use the p-value for estimating the magnitude of your study result, or, subsequently, to conclude from differences in p-values that one study result is better than the other. A small p-value may not only indicate a large study effect but also a large sample size and a small spread in the data. Indeed, with very large study samples it is almost impossible to avoid finding significant p-values that are clinically utterly irrelevant. Statisticians, therefore, have an aversion from very large samples. Also a large spread in the data will cause large and insignificant p-values even with large study results.

7   Renewed Interpretations of P-Values, Little Difference Between P = 0.060 and P = 0.040

H0 is currently less dogmatically rejected, because we believe that such practice mistakenly attempts to express certainty of statistical evidence in the data. If the H0 is rejected, it is also no longer concluded that there is no difference in the data. Instead, we increasingly believe that there is actually little difference between p = 0.06 and p = 0.04. Like with business statistics clinicians now have the option to use p-values for an additional purpose, i.e., for making decisions about the risks they are willing to take.

Also an advantage of the exact p-value approach is the possibility of more refined conclusions from the research: instead of concluding significantly yes/no,

Table 6.1 The famous t-table as computed without the help of a computer in the 1930s by data tightening techniques

T-Table: v = degrees of freedom for t-variable, Q = area under the curve right from the corresponding t-value, $2Q$ tests both right and left end of the total area under the curve

v	Q = 0.4	0.25	0.1	0.05	0.025	0.01	0.005	0.001
	2Q = 0.8	0.5	0.2	0.1	0.05	0.02	0.01	0.002
1	0.325	1.000	3.078	6.314	12.706	31.821	63.657	318.31
2	.289	0.816	1.886	2.920	4.303	6.965	9.925	22.326
3	.277	.765	1.638	2.353	3.182	4.547	5.841	10.213
4	.171	.741	1.533	2.132	2.776	3.747	4.604	7.173
5	0.267	0.727	1.476	2.015	2.571	3.365	4.032	5.893
6	.265	.718	1.440	1.943	2.447	3.143	3.707	5.208
7	.263	.711	1.415	1.895	2.365	2.998	3.499	4.785
8	.262	.706	1.397	1.860	2.306	2.896	3.355	4.501
9	.261	.703	1.383	1.833	2.262	2.821	3.250	4.297
10	0.261	0.700	1.372	1.812	2.228	2.764	3.169	4.144
11	.269	.697	1.363	1.796	2.201	2.718	3.106	4.025
12	.269	.695	1.356	1.782	2.179	2.681	3.055	3.930
13	.259	.694	1.350	1.771	2.160	2.650	3.012	3.852
14	.258	.692	1.345	1.761	2.145	2.624	2.977	3.787
15	0.258	0.691	1.341	1.753	2.131	2.602	2.947	3.733
16	.258	.690	1.337	1.746	2.120	2.583	2.921	3.686
17	.257	.689	1.333	1.740	2.110	2.567	2.898	3.646
18	.257	688	1.330	1.734	2.101	2.552	2.878	3.610
19	.257	.688	1.328	1.729	2.093	2.539	2.861	3.579
20	0.257	0.687	1.325	1.725	2.086	2.528	2.845	3.552
21	.257	.686	1.323	1.721	2.080	2.518	2.831	3.527
22	.256	.686	1.321	1.717	2.074	2.508	2.819	3.505
23	.256	.685	1.319	1.714	2.069	2.600	2.807	3.485
24	.256	.685	1.318	1.711	2.064	2.492	2.797	3.467
25	0.256	0.684	1,316	1.708	2.060	2.485	2.787	3.450
26	.256	.654	1,315	1.706	2.056	2.479	2.779	3.435
27	.256	.684	1,314	1.701	2.052	2.473	2.771	3.421
28	.256	.683	1,313	1.701	2.048	2.467	2.763	3.408
29	.256	.683	1,311	1.699	2.045	2.462	2.756	3.396
30	0.256	0.683	1.310	1.697	2.042	2.457	2.750	3.385
40	.255	.681	1.303	1.684	2.021	2.423	2.704	3.307
60	.254	.679	1.296	1.671	2.000	2.390	2.660	3.232
120	.254	.677	1.289	1.658	1.950	2.358	2.617	3.160
∞	.253	.674	1.282	1.645	1.960	2.326	2.576	3.090

we are able to consider levels of probabilities from very likely to be true, to very likely to be untrue [12]. The p-value which ranges from 0.0 to 1.0 summarizes the evidence in the data about H0. A large p-value such as 0.55 or 0.78 indicates that the observed data would not be unusual if H0 were true. A small p-value such as 0.001 denotes that these data would be very doubtful if H0 were true. This provides strong support against H0. In such instances results are said to be significant at the 0.001 level, indicating that getting a result of this size might occur only 1 out of 1,000 times.

Exact p-values are also increasingly used for comparing different levels of significance. The drawback of this approach is that sampled frequency distributions are approximations, and that it can be mathematically shown that exactly calculated p-values are rather inaccurate [13]. However, this drawback is outweighed by the advantages of knowing the p-values especially when it gets to extremes [14].

8   The Real Meaning of Very Large P-Values Like P > 0.950

Let us assume that in a Mendelian experiment the expected ratio of yellow-peas/green-peas = 1/1. A highly representative random sample of n = 100 might consist of 50 yellow and 50 green peas. However, the larger the sample the smaller the chance to find exactly 50/50. The chance of exactly 5,000 yellow/5,000 green peas or even the chance of a result very close to this result is, due to large variability in biological processes, almost certainly zero.

Statistical distributions like the chi-square distribution can account for this lack of perfection in experimental data sampling, and provide exact probability levels of finding results close to "expected". Chi-squares curves are skewed curves with a lengthy right-end (Fig. 6.2).

We reject the null-hypothesis of no difference between "expected and observed", if the area under curve (AUC) on the right side of the calculated chi-square value is <5 % of the total AUC. Chi-square curves do, however, also have a short left-end which ends with a chi-square value of zero. If the chi-square value calculated from our data is close to zero, the left AUC will get smaller and smaller, and as it becomes <5 % of the total AUC, we are equally justified not to accept the null hypothesis as we are with large chi-square values. E.g., in a sample of 10,000 peas, you might find 4,997 yellow and 5,003 green peas. Are these data representative for a population of 1/1 yellow/green peas? In this example a chi-square value of $<3.9 \ 10^{-3}$ indicates that the left AUC is <5 % and, so, we have a probability <5 % to find it (Table 6.2) [15].

Chi-square value is calculated according to:

$$\text{(Observed yellow} - \text{Expected yellow)}^2 = (4997 - 5000)^2 : 5000 \text{ to standardize} = 1.8 \ 10^{-3}$$
$$\text{(Observed green} - \text{Expected green)}^2 = (5003 - 5000)^2 : 5000 \text{ to standardize} = 1.8 \ 10^{-3}$$
$$\text{chi} - \text{square (1 degree of freedom)} = 3.6 \ 10^{-3}$$

This result is smaller than $3.9 \ 10^{-3}$ and, thus, it is so close to what was expected that we can only conclude that we have <5 % probability to find it. We have to scrutinize these results, and must consider and examine the possibility of

Fig. 6.2 Probability of
finding χ^2 value >3.841 is
<0.05, so is probability of
finding a χ^2 value <0.0039.
AUC area under the curve,
df degree of freedom

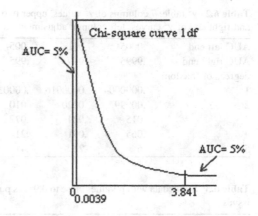

inadequate data improvement. The above example is actually based on some true historic facts (Mendel indeed improved his data) [16].

We searched for main endpoint p-values close to 0.95 in randomized controlled trials published in recent issues of the Lancet and the New England Journal of Medicine, and found four studies [17–20]. Table 6.3 gives a summary. All of these studies aimed at demonstrating similarities rather than differences. Indeed, as can be observed, proportions of patients with events in the treatment and control groups were very similar. E.g., the percentages in treatment and control groups of patients with sepsis were 1.3 and 1.3 % (study 1, Table 6.3), and of patients with cardio-vascular events 79.2 and 79.8 % (study 5, Table 6.3). The investigators of the studies calculated p-values from $p > 0.94$ to $p > 0.995$, which, according to the chi-square table (Table 6.2), would provide left-end p-values between ≤ 0.06 and ≤ 0.005. This would mean, that, for whatever reason, these data were probably not completely random. Unwarranted exclusion of, otherwise, appropriate outliers is one of the possible explanations.

9   The Real Meaning of Very Small P-Values Like P < 0.0001

Statistics gives no certainties, only chances. A generally accepted concept is "the smaller the p-value the better reliable the results". This is not entirely true with current randomized controlled trials. First, randomized controlled trials are designed to test small differences. A randomized controlled trial with major differences between old and new treatment is unethical because half of the patients have been given an inferior treatment.

Second, they are designed to confirm prior evidence. For that purpose, their sample size is carefully calculated. Not only too small but also too large a sample size is considered unethical and unscientific, because negative studies have to be repeated and a potentially inferior treatment should not be given to too many

Table 6.2 χ^2 table: 7 columns of χ^2 values, upper two rows areas under the curve (AUCs) of left and right end of χ^2 curves, left column: adjustments for degrees of freedom (dfs)

AUC left end	.0005	.001	.005	.01	.025	.05	.10
AUC right end	.9995	.999	.995	.99	.975	.95	.90
degrees of freedom							
1	.0000004	.0000016	.000039	.00016	.00091	.0039	.016
2	.00099	.0020	.010	.020	.051	.10	.21
3	.015	.024	.072	.12	.22	.35	.58
4	.065	.091	.21	.30	.48	.71	1.06
5	.6	.21	.41	.55	.83	1.154	1.61

Table 6.3 Study data with p-values close to 0.95, as published in recent Lancet and N Engl J Med issues

Result (numbers)	Results (%)	Sample size requirement	Alpha-level	P-values
Ref. [17] 107/6264 vs. 107/6262	1.7 vs. 1.7	Yes	0.05	>0.995
Ref. [18] 88/965 vs. 84/941	9.1 vs. 8.9	Yes	0.05	>0.95
Ref. [18] 13/965 vs. 12/941	1.3 vs. 1.3	Yes	0.05	>0.95
Ref. [19] 214/1338 vs. 319/2319	15.9 vs. 13.8	Yes	0.05	>0.99
Ref. [20] 285/360 vs. 1087/1363	79.2 vs. 79.8	Yes	0.05	>0.94

1. Proportions of patients with heart infarction in patients with diastolic blood pressure 80 < . . . < 85 vs. < 80 mmHg
2. Proportion of patients with arrhythmias in patients with standard perioperative treatment vs. Swann-Ganz catheter-guided perioperative treatment
3. Proportion of patients with sepsis in patients with standard perioperative treatment vs. Swann-Ganz catheter-guided perioperative treatment
4. Proportions of patients with cardiovascular events in patients with LDL-cholesterol, <3.5 mmol/l vs. 3.5 < . . . < 4.5 mmol/l
5. Proportions of patients with cardiovascular events in patients with LDL-cholesterol <2.6 mmol/l vs. >3.4 mmol/l. *Alpha* type I error, *vs.* versus

patients. Often in the study protocol a statistical power of 80 % is agreed, corresponding with a p-value of approximately 0.01.

The ultimate p-value may then be a bit larger or smaller. However a p-value of >0.05 will be rarely observed, because current clinical trials are confirmational and, therefore, rarely negative. Also a p-value much smaller than 0.01 will be rarely observed, because it would indicate that either the power assessment was inadequate (the study is overpowered) or the data have been artificially improved. With p = 0.0001 we have a peculiar situation. In this situation the actual data can not only reject the null-hypothesis, but also the hypothesis of significantly better Thus, a p-value <0.0001, if the power was set at 80 %, does not completely confirm its prior expectations and must be scrutinized for data improvement (Fig. 6.3).

Table 6.4 gives an overview of five published studies with main endpoint p-values <0.0001 [21–24]. All of these studies were published in the first 6 issues of the 1992 volume of the New England Journal of Medicine. It is remarkable that so many overpowered studies were published within 6 subsequent months of a

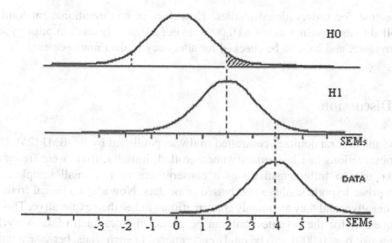

Fig. 6.3 Null-hypothesis (H0), hypothesis of significantly better (H1), and actual data distribution (DATA) of an example of experimental data with n = 120 and mean = 3.90 SEMs and a t-distributed frequency distribution. The actual data can not only reject H0 (t = 3.90, p = 0.0001), but also H1 (t = 1.95, p = 0.05). This would mean that not only H0 but also H1 is untrue. *SEM* standard error of the mean

Table 6.4 Study data with p-values as low as <0.0001, published in the first 6 issues of the 1992 volume of the N Engl J Med

Result	Sample size requirement	Alpha-level	P-values
Ref. [21] +0.5 vs. +2.1 %	Yes	0.05	<0.0001
Ref. [21] −2.8 vs. +1.8 %	Yes	0.05	<0.0001
Ref. [22] 11 vs. 19 %	No	0.05	<0.0001
Ref. [23] r = −0.53	No	0.05	<0.0001
Ref. [24] 213 vs. 69	No	0.05	<0.0001

In the past 4 years p-values smaller than p < 0.001 were never published in this journal
1. Duration exercise in patients after medical therapy vs. percutaneous coronary angioplasty
2. Maximal double product (systolic blood pressure times heart rate) during exercise in patients after medical treatment vs. percutaneous coronary angioplasty
3. Erythromycin resistance throat swabs vs. pus samples
4. Correlation between reduction of epidermal pigmentation during treatment and baseline amount of pigmentation
5. Adverse reactions of high vs. non-high osmolality agents during cardiac catheterization. *Alpha* type I error, *vs.* versus

single volume, while the same journal published not any study with p-values below 0.001 in the past 4 years' full volumes. We do not know why, but this may be due to the journal's policy not to accept studies with very low p-values anymore. In contrast, many other journals including the Lancet, Circulation, BMJ, abound with extremely low p-values. It is obvious that these journals still believe in the concept "the lower the p-value, the better reliable the research". The concept may still be true for observational studies. However, in confirmational randomized controlled trials, p-values as low as 0.0001 do not adequately confirm prior hypotheses anymore, and have to be checked for adequacy of data management.

10   Discussion

In 1948 the first randomized controlled trial was published by the BMJ [25]. Until then, observations had been mainly uncontrolled. Initially, trials were frequently negative due to little sensitivity as a consequence of too small samples, and inappropriate hypotheses based on biased prior data. Nowadays, clinical trials are rarely negative, and they are mainly confirmational rather than explorative. This has consequences for the p-values that can be expected from such trials. Very low p-values like $p < 0.0001$ will be rarely encountered in such trials, because it would mean that the study was overpowered and should have had a smaller sample size. Also very large p-values like $p > 0.95$ will be rare, because they would indicate similarities closer than compatible with a normal distribution of random data samples.

We should emphasize that the above-mentioned interpretation of very low/high p-values is only true within the context of randomized controlled trials. E.g., unrandomized observational data can easily produce very low and very high p-values, and there is nothing wrong with that. Also the above interpretation is untrue in clinical trials that test multiple endpoints rather than a single main endpoint or a single composite endpoint. Clinical trials testing multiple rather than single endpoints, often do so for the purpose of answering a single question, e.g., the benefit of health of a new drug may be estimated by mortality in addition to various morbidity variables. If investigators test many times, they are apt to find differences, e.g., 5 % of the time, but this may not be due to significant effects but rather to chance. In this situation, one should informally integrate all of the data before reaching conclusions, and look for the trends in the data without judging one or two low p-values, among otherwise high p-values, as proof.

In the present chapter, for the assessment of high p-values, the chi-square test is used, while for the assessment of low p-values the t-test is used. Both tests are, however, closely related to one another, and like other statistical tests, including the F-test, regression analysis, and other tests based on normal distributions. The conclusions drawn from our assessments are, therefore, equally true for alternative statistical tests and data.

We should add that the nominal p-values have to be interpreted with caution in case of multiple testing. A not yet mentioned but straightforward way to correct this is to calculate an E-value, i.e. the product of the p-value and the number of tests.

P-values <0.0001 will be rarely encountered in randomized controlled clinical trials, because it would mean that the study is overpowered and should have had a smaller sample size. Also p-values >0.95 will be rare, because they would indicate similarities closer than compatible with a normal distribution of random samples.

It would seem appropriate, therefore, to require investigators to explain such results, and to consider rejecting the research involved. So far, in randomized controlled trials the null-hypothesis is generally rejected at $p < 0.05$. Maybe, we should consider rejecting the entire study if the main endpoint p-values are >0.95 or <0.0001.

The concept of the p-value is notoriously poorly understood. Some physicians even comfortably think that the p-value is a measure of effect [26]. When asked whether a drug treatment worked, their typical answer would be: "Well, p is less than 0.05, so I guess it did". The more knowledgeable among us know that p stands for chance (probability = p), and that there must be risks of errors. The current paper reviews the standard as well as renewed interpretations of the p-values, and was written for physicians accepting statistical reasoning as a required condition for an adequate assessment of the benefits and limitations of evidence-based medicine.

Additional points must be considered when interpreting the p-values. In the first place, the interpretation of low p-values is different in studies that test multiple endpoints rather than a single main endpoint or a single composite endpoint. Studies testing multiple rather than single endpoints, often do so for the purpose of answering a single question, e.g., the benefit of health of a new drug may be estimated by mortality in addition to various morbidity variables. If investigators test many times, they are apt to find differences, e.g., 5 % of the time, but this may not be due to significant effects but rather to chance. In this situation, one should informally integrate all of the data before reaching conclusions, and look for the trends in the data without judging one or two low p-values, among otherwise high p-values, as proof.

Special attention in this respect deserves the issue of multiple low-powered studies. One might consider this situation to be similar to the above one, and conclude that such studies be similarly integrated. Actually, this is one of the concepts of the method of meta-analysis. Second, the point of one sided testing versus two-sided testing must be considered. Studies testing both ends of a normal frequency distribution have twice the chance of finding a significant difference compared to those testing only one end. If our research assesses whether there is any difference in the data, no matter in what direction, either the positive or the negative one, then we have a two-sided design and the p-values must doubled. It is then, consequently, harder to obtain a low p-value.

Recommendations regarding the interpretation of main-endpoint-study p-values either two-sided or not, include the following.

11 Conclusions

1. $P < 0.05$ gives a conditional probability: H0 can be rejected on the limitations/ assumptions that (1) we have up to 5 % chance of a type I error of finding a difference where there is none, (2) we have 50 % chance of a type II error of finding no difference where there is one, (3) the data are normally distributed,

(4) they follow exactly the same distribution as that of the population from which the sample was taken.

2. A common misunderstanding is the concept that the p-value is actually the chance that H0 is true, and, consequently that a $p > 0.05$ indicates a significant similarity in the data. $P > 0.05$ may, indeed, indicate similarity. However, also a study-sample too small or study design inadequate to detect the difference must be considered.

3. An advantage of the exact p-values is the possibility of more refined conclusions from the research: instead of concluding significantly yes/no, we are able to consider levels of probabilities from very likely to be true, to very likely to be untrue.

4. $P > 0.95$ suggests that the observed data are closer to expectation than compatible with a Gaussian frequency distribution, and such results must, therefore, be scrutinized.

5. A $p < 0.0001$, if power was set at 80 %, does not completely confirm the prior expectations of the power assessment. Therefore, such results must be scrutinized.

6. The p-values tell us the chance of making a type I error of finding a difference where there is none. In the 1970s exact p-values were laborious to calculate, and they were, generally, approximated from statistical tables, in the form of $p < 0.01$ or $0.05 < p < 0.10$ etc. In the past decades with the advent of computers it became easy to calculate exact p-values such as 0.840 or 0.007. The cut-off p-values have not been completely abandoned, but broader attention is given to the interpretation of the exact p-values.

References

1. SAS Statistical Software (2013) www.sas.com. 2 Sept 2013
2. SPSS Statistical Software (2013) www.spss.com. 2 Sept 2013
3. S-plus Statistical Software (2013) www.splus.com. 2 Sept 2013
4. Stata Statistical Software (2013) www.stata.com. 2 Sept 2013
5. P Value Calculator (2013) http://Graphpad.com/quickcalcs/PValue.1.cfm. 30 June 2013
6. Z Score to P Value Calculator (2013) Easycalculation.com>Statistics. 30 June 2013
7. Free p-Value Calculation for an F-test (2013) www.danielsoper.com>StatisticsCalculators. 30 June 2013
8. Levin RI, Rubin DS (1998) P-value. In: Levin RI, Rubin DS (eds) Statistics for management. Prentice-Hall, Upper Saddle River, NJ, USA, pp 485–496
9. Utts JM (1999) P-value. In: Utts JM (ed) Seeing through statistics. Duxbury Press, Detroit, pp 375–386
10. Cleophas TJ, Zwinderman AH, Cleophas AF (2004) P-values. Review. Am J Ther 11:317–322
11. Cleophas TJ, Zwinderman AH, Cleophas AF (2004) P-values, beware of the extremes. Clin Chem Lab Med 42:300–305
12. Michelson S, Schofield T (1996) P-values as conditional probabilities. In: Michelson S, Schofield T (eds) The biostatistics cookbook. Kluwer Academic Publishers, Boston, pp 46–58
13. Petrie A, Sabin C (2000) Explanation of p-values. In: Petrie A, Sabin C (eds) Medical statistics at glance. Blackwell Science, Oxford, pp 42–45

14. Matthews DE, Farewel VT (1996) P-value. In: Matthews DE, Farewell VT (eds) Using and understanding medical statistics. Karger, New York, pp 15–18
15. Riffenburgh RH (1999) P-values. In: Riffenburgh RH (ed) Statistics in medicine. Academic Press, San Diego, pp 95–96, 105–106
16. Cleophas TJ, Cleophas GM (2001) Sponsored research and continuing medical education. JAMA 286:302–304
17. Hansson L, Zanchetti A, Carruthers SG, Dahlof B, Elmfeldt D, Julius S et al, for the HOT Study Group (1998) Effects of intensive blood pressure lowering and low-dose aspirin in patients with hypertension: principal results of the Hypertension Optimal Treatment (HOT) randomised trial. Lancet 351:1755–1762
18. Sandham JD, Hull RD, Brand RF, Knox L, Pineo GF, Doig CJ et al, for the Canadian Critical Care Clinical Trials Group (2003) A randomized, controlled trial of the use of pulmonary-artery catheters in high-risk surgical patients. N Engl J Med 348:5–14
19. LIPID Study Group (2002) Long-term effectiveness and safety of pravastatin in 9014 patients with coronary heart disease and average cholesterol concentrations: the LIPID trial follow-up. Lancet 359:1379–1387
20. Heart Protection Study Collaborative Group (2002) MRC/BHF Heart Protection Study of cholesterol lowering with simvastatin in 20536 high-risk individuals: a randomised placebo-controlled trial. Lancet 360:7–22
21. Parisi AF, Folland ED, Hartigan P, on behalf of the Veterans Affairs ACME Investigators (1992) A comparison of angioplasty with medical therapy in the treatment of single-vessel coronary artery disease. N Engl J Med 326:10–16
22. Seppälä H, Nissinen A, Järvinen H, Huovinen S, Henrikson T, Herva E et al (1992) Resistance to erythromycin in group A streptococci. N Engl J Med 326:292–297
23. Rafal ES, Griffiths CE, Ditre CM, Finkel LJ, Hamilton TA, Ellis CN et al (1992) Topical retinoin treatment for liver spots associated with photodamage. N Engl J Med 326:368–374
24. Barrett BJ, Parfrey PS, Vavasour HM, O'Dea F, Kent G, Stone E (1992) A comparison of nonionic, low-osmolality radiocontrast agents with ionic, high-osmolality agents during cardiac catheterization. N Engl J Med 326:431–436
25. Medical Research Council (1948) Streptomycin treatment of pulmonary tuberculosis. Br Med J 2:769–782
26. Motulsky H (1995) P-values, definition and common misinterpretations. In: Motulsky H (ed) Intuitive biostatistics. Oxford University Press, New York, pp 96–97

Chapter 7
Probit Regression

1 Summary

1.1 Background

The term multivariate analysis indicates the analysis of a study with multiple outcome variables. No standard method for multiple binary outcome variables is available, while in clinical research, often multiple events/outcomes are the outcome of a study.

1.2 Objective

To asses the efficiency of multivariate probit analysis for the purpose.

1.3 Methods

A real data example of the effect of physicians' age on lifestyle advise was used. A stepwise analysis is given. Also post hoc analyses are done.

1.4 Results

Unlike binary logistic regressions, a multivariate probit analysis provided very significant results with a log likelihood value of -15.96 and a p-value of 0.0001.

T.J. Cleophas and A.H. Zwinderman, *Machine Learning in Medicine: Part Three*, DOI 10.1007/978-94-007-7869-6_7, © Springer Science+Business Media Dordrecht 2013

1.5   Conclusions

1. In clinical research event analysis is relevant, and, often, more than a single event/outcome value is the subject of study.
2. Unfortunately, no standard method for simultaneous analysis of multiple events/ outcomes is available.
3. Multivariate probit analysis included in the statistical program of STATA and traditionally used in social science, could be used for the purpose of multiple event/outcome analysis of clinical research data.
4. It is a safe alternative to multivariate logistic regression.
5. In case of a significant multivariate probit regression, post hoc analysis can be performed in the usual way by binary logistic models to find out which outcome is more important, but post hoc tests need not necessarily be significant.
6. Probit analysis is adequate for multivariate data with binary outcomes and performs better than multivariate logistic regression does.

2   Introduction

Linear, logistic, and Cox regressions are examples of analysis methods with a single outcome variable. If these methods included multiple predictors variables (otherwise called exposure variables or x-variables), they are sometimes called multivariate methods. But this is not correct, because the term multivariate analysis refers to the simultaneous analysis of more than a single *outcome* variable. A more adequate term for the analysis of multiple predictors variables is "multivariable or multiple variables analysis".

In clinical research often multiple outcomes variables are being assessed. E.g., in a study of physicians' reluctance to provide life style advise the outcome variables may be different forms of life style advise given and the predictor variable may be the physicians' age or any other physicians' characteristic. If the outcome variables are continuous like scores, then path analysis or multiple analysis of variance are adequate [1]. If, however, the outcome variables are binary, like a smoking advise and a weight reduction advise given or not, then a multivariate method for binary outcomes is required.

For univariate analyses with binary outcome variables logistic regression is adequate. A problem with logistic regression with multiple outcome variables is that after iteration (= computer program for finding the largest log likelihood ratio for fitting the data) the results often do not converse, i.e., a best log likelihood ratio is not established. This is due to insufficient data size, inadequate data, or non quadratic data patterns. A better alternative for that purpose is probit modeling. This may sound incomprehensible, but the dependent variable of logistic regression (the log odds of responding) is closely related to log probit (probit is the z-value corresponding to its area under curve value of the normal distribution). It can be shown that log odds of responding = logit $\approx (\pi/\sqrt{3}) \times$ probit [2]. Multivariate probit analysis is not available in SPSS [3] and we will use the statistical software of the program Stata (STATA 10) [4].

Probit analysis, apart from its use in biological assays, particularly the death analysis of insects exposed to toxics, is currently mainly used in social science [2].

Medical investigators are often involved in event analysis. This chapter was written to explain probit analysis as a welcome method for analyzing clinical studies with more than a single event as outcome. A real data example was used, and step-by-step analyses are given, including post hoc analyses.

3 Example

An example is given of the effect of the physicians' age (x) on their inclination to prescribe life style treatments (1) non smoking advise (0 = no, 1 = yes) and (2) weight reduction advise (0 = no, 1 = yes), (y and z), (Var = variable).

Var	Var	Var
(x)	(y)	(z)
42.7	0	0
47.6	0	0
36.4	0	0
49.0	0	0
49.0	0	1
55.3	0	1
57.4	0	1
63.0	0	1
27.3	0	1
53.2	1	0
54.6	1	0
32.9	1	0

We can input the data in STATA statistical software [4] directly from an SPSS data file with the commands (the data file entitled "chap7probit.sav" is on the internet at extras.springer.com):

Input x y z....input values....end....List....Statistics....binary outcomes....Bivariate probit regression....dependent variable 1 y....dependent variable 2 z.....independent variables x..... OK.

Table 7.1 shows that physicians' age is significant predictor of both prescribing non smoking and weight reduction advise with a log likelihood value of −15.96 and a p-value of 0.0001. In order to find out which is the most significant outcome, simple binary logistic regression can be performed using physicians' ages as predictor and the non drug treatments as separate outcomes.

Table 7.1 According to the underneath analysis the probit regression in STATA shows that indeed physicians' age is significant predictor of both prescribing non smoking and weight reduction advise

STATA
Probit var 3 var 2 var 1
Fitting comparison equation 1:
Iteration 0: log likelihood = −8.3177662
Fitting comparison equation 2:
Iteration 0: log likelihood = −8.3177662
Comparison: log likelihood = −16.635532
Fitting full model:
Iteration 0: log likelihood = −16.635532
Iteration 1: log likelihood = −15.9573
Iteration 2: log likelihood = −15.955936
Iteration 3: log likelihood = −15.955936

Bivariate probit regression

Number of observations = 12
Wald chi2 (2) = 0.00
Prob > chi2 = 1.0000

Log likelihood = −15.955936
  2 log likelihood ratio = 31.911872
   P < 0.000

Table 7.2 Binary logistic regression in SPSS with non smoking advise as outcome shows that the physicians' age is not a significant predictor

Variables in the equation		B	S.E.	Wald	df	Sig.	Exp(B)
Step 1[a]	Physician age	−,006	,065	,008	1	,927	,994
	Constant	−,819	3,121	,069	1	,793	,441

[a]Variable(s) entered on step 1: physician age

We will use SPSS statistical software for the purpose.

Command: Analyze....Regression....Binary Logistic....Dependent: enter smoking advise....Covariate: enter physicians' age....OK.

The outcome sheets show that the physicians' age is not a significant predictor (Table 7.2). A similar binary logistic regression with weight reduction advise as outcome is again not statistically significant (Table 7.3).

After Bonferroni adjustment of the rejection p-value (p = 0.05 × 2/3 (3−1) = 0.0166, see Chap. 3, p. 24) we will still find a very significant multivariate p-value of two very insignificant p-values for the post hoc tests. The overall conclusion from the analyses would be that the physicians' age, although a very significant predictor of the combination "smoking advise" and "weight reduction advise" is not a significant predictor of either of the variables separately. How is that possible? If we look at the data, we will observe that 7 physicians are under 50 years and 5 are older than 50 years. In the younger group only 3/7 (43 %) gives at least one lifestyle advise, while in the older group 5/5 (100 %) gives at least one

Table 7.3 Binary logistic regression in SPSS with weight reduction advise as outcome shows that the physicians' age is not a significant predictor

Variables in the equation

		B	S.E.	Wald	df	Sig.	Exp(B)
Step 1[a]	Physician age	,054	,064	,714	1	,398	1,055
	Constant	−2,913	3,149	,856	1	,355	,54

[a]Variable(s) entered on step 1: physician age

lifestyle advise. Despite the negative univariate analyses, the difference between older and younger physicians may be real. In order to find further support for that, a chi-square test is performed.

	Lifestyle advise	
	yes	no
Under 50	3	4
Over 50	5	0

$$\text{The chi-square value} = \frac{(3 \times 0 - 4 \times 5)^2 \times (3 + 4 + 0 + 5)}{(3 + 5)(4 + 0)(3 + 4)(5 + 0)} = 4.3,$$

With 1 degree of freedom this would mean that $p < 0.05$, and, thus, that there is, indeed, a significant difference between the older than younger physicians. This supports that the multivariate analysis is adequate and supports that the difference is clinically relevant.

4 Discussion

Multivariate analysis is not adequate as a method for explorative research, that is research with little prior hypothesis if any. This is so, because it has generally weak statistical power, as it is a complex method taken multiple variations simultaneously into account. In contrast, for confirmative research, that is research with a sound prior hypothesis, particularly if it is complex, multivariate analysis is appropriate, and can reveal otherwise hidden effects. The example gives an example of the effects of age on two outcomes, (1) non smoking advise, weight reduction advise. This small trial is unable to demonstrate significant univariate effects of physicians' age on lifestyle advise given. However, when more than a single lifestyle advise is tested simultaneously a very significant effect is observed. Other advantages of multivariate analysis include the following.

1. It prevents the type I error from being inflated, because, instead of multiple testing, a single overall test is performed.
2. It is the only method that takes interactions between dependent variables in relationship with a predictor into account.
3. It can sometimes detect subgroup properties and includes them in the analysis, and sometimes demonstrates otherwise underpowered effects.

Clinical data with multiple binary outcomes like events is commonly observed, and the traditional logistic regression for that purpose requires multiple separate tests and Bonferroni adjustments. In addition, other advantages, as mentioned above, are not covered. A multivariate analysis using logistic regression is often impossible, as explained in the introduction section. Fortunately, multivariate probit regression, although not available in SPSS, is a safe alternative for multivariate logistic regression, and it is available in Stata and other software programs. In case of a significant multivariate probit regression, post hoc analysis can be performed in the usual way by binary logistic models to find out which of the outcome is more important, but, as shown, the post hoc tests need not necessarily be significant.

5 Conclusions

1. In clinical research event analysis is relevant, and, often, more than a single event is the subject of study.
2. Unfortunately, no standard method for simultaneous analysis of multiple events is available.
3. Multivariate probit analysis included in the statistical program of STATA and traditionally used in social science, could be used for the purpose of multiple event analysis in clinical research.
4. It is a safe alternative to multivariate logistic regression.
5. In case of a significant multivariate probit regression, post hoc analysis can be performed in the usual way by binary logistic models to find out which of the outcome is more important, but post hoc tests need not necessarily be significant.

References

1. Cleophas TJ, Zwinderman AH (2012) Multivariate analysis, chapter 25. In: Cleophas TJ, Zwinderman AH (eds) Statistics applied to clinical studies, 5th edn. Springer, Heidelberg, pp 289–299
2. Hagle T (2014) Probit analysis. In: Lewis-Beck MS, Bryman A, Liao's TF (eds) SAGE encyclopedia of social sciences. SAGE, New York, pp 710–720. doi:10.4135/97814122950589
3. SPSS Statistical Software (2013) www.spss.com. 2 Sept 2013
4. STATA Statistical Software (2013) www.stata.com. 2 Sept 2013

Chapter 8
Over-Dispersion

1 Summary

1.1 Background

Over-dispersion depicts the phenomenon that the spread in the data is wider than compatible with Gaussian modeling. The phenomenon may occur both with continuous and discrete data, although more commonly with discrete data.

1.2 Objective

To assess whether non-mathematicians are able to adjust over-dispersion in their data.

1.3 Methods

Two binary data examples are given. One is analyzed without, the other with special help from SPSS statistical software.

1.4 Results

In a clinical trial of b-blockers and calcium channel blockers the probability of responding was unchanged after adjustment for over-dispersion but the 95 % confidence interval rose from 0.31–0.42 to 0.28–0.45. In a study of predictors of

T.J. Cleophas and A.H. Zwinderman, *Machine Learning in Medicine: Part Three*,   69
DOI 10.1007/978-94-007-7869-6_8, © Springer Science+Business Media Dordrecht 2013

torsades de pointes the sensitivity of testing treatment efficacy fell from 0.0001 to 0.007. Psychological and social scores were insignificant after adjustment for over-dispersion, which was in agreement with the investigators' prior hypotheses.

1.5   Conclusions

1. Over-dispersion means that the spread in the data is wider than compatible with Gaussian modeling. Traditional statistical tests overestimate the precision of over-dispersed data, meaning that the calculated p-values are too small, and the conclusion of a significant effect is erroneously made.
2. Over-dispersion is more commonly observed with binary data than it is with continuous data.
3. Several tests are available but Pearson goodness of fit test is often used to assess and adjust over-dispersion.
4. For binary data SPSS offers a Poisson model adjusted for over-dispersion.
5. With large differences in the data, the presence of over-dispersion should be assessed and adjusted.
6. Non-mathematicians are able to do so either with or without the help of SPSS tests especially developed for the purpose.

2   Introduction

Over-dispersion depicts the phenomenon that the spread in the data is wider than compatible with Gaussian modeling [1]. Traditional statistical tests overestimate the precision of over-dispersed data, meaning that the calculated p-values are too small, and the conclusion of a significant effect is erroneously being made [2]. The issue of over-dispersion, although recognized as a potential problem in real world data already in 1953 by Ronald Fisher [3], the famous London UK statistician and inventor of ANOVA (analysis of variance), has not yet been routinely accounted or assessed in clinical research. Fortunately, in recent research it is increasingly being recognized as a fundamental aspect of describing sampled data [4]. Over-dispersion may occur both with continuous and binary data, although more commonly with the latter [5]. To date statistical software programs do not routinely include tests for over-dispersion, and, so, investigators have to take care and make their own assessments prior to the analysis [2]. Also, for binary data a method for adjusting over-dispersion is now available in SPSS in the module Generalized linear mixed effects [6]. The current chapter gives some real and hypothesized examples to demonstrate how it should be implemented in data analyses. Also an example with stepwise analyses in SPSS is given for the benefit of investigators.

3   Some Theory

Figure 8.1 gives a graph of our trial data with the individual data on the x-axis and "how often" on the y-axis. The wide curve summarizes the mean and the spread pattern of our trial data. In predictive research we are, however, generally more interested in the means and spread of many future trials similar to our trial than that of our trial. This is assessed by the narrow curve. It summarizes the means of many trials similar to ours. Why so? This is, because our trial is representative of the target population, and, if we would repeat the trial, the result would be approximately the same.

The summary of the means of many trials is narrower, and has less outliers than the individual data. This is so, because it has sems (standard errors of the means) instead of standard deviations on the x-axis, and sem $= sd/\sqrt{n}$. Gauss [7], the German mathematician in 1800, found out that in many experimental situations the narrow curve has a reproducible pattern with in the interval mean ± 1 sem 70 % of the trials and in the interval mean ± 2 sems 95 % of the trials. He recommended that the reproducible pattern was effective for testing statistical hypotheses

> 1/no difference new and old,
> 2/real difference,
> 3/new worse than old,
> 4/two treatments equivalent etc.

However, why should the overall mean of many trials similar to our trial have exactly the same mean as our calculated mean. This would be, particularly, untrue, if trials were over-dispersed, otherwise called heterogeneous, and the overall mean could, then, better be presented by a range of means. Consequently, a single sem-curve would need to be replaced with a range of sem-curves, as the traditional

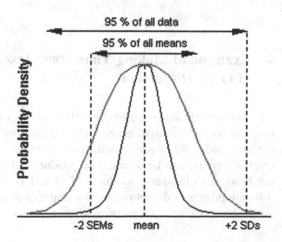

Fig. 8.1 Simple Gaussian
frequency distribution
curves to summarize a trial
data file

sem-curve for describing our data and testing our hypotheses would be too narrow. Over-dispersion may have been a negligible problem in the time of Gauss who used mainly continuous data. However, in current research binary data (event data) are increasingly used, and the phenomenon of over-dispersion is, particularly, common with such data. When summarizing binary data, the proportion (p) of events is used to indicate the mean result. The standard deviation of a proportion is given by p (1 − p), is, thus, entirely determined by the magnitude of p. In practice, the sequences in binary sampling are often dependent on one another, and this is likely to produce covariances, and, consequently, over-dispersion in the data. The equation p(1 − p), then, underestimates the true spread in the data.

In order to assess this problem, it would make sense to first perform a test for heterogeneity in your data, like the heterogeneity test used in meta-analyses of multiple comparable studies, and only accept a single overall mean, if heterogeneity can be rejected. Several tests are available, but the Pearson goodness of fit test [8] is often used. It assumes that multiple proportions of events from similar studies follow a Gaussian pattern. The area under the curve of a Gaussian curve is split into 5 equiprobable intervals of 20 % each, and we expect approximately 1/5 of the proportions per interval. If the observed numbers in each interval is significantly different from the expected, the data will be over-dispersed, and the magnitude of the test statistic used here (a chi-square value) is a measure for the degree of over-dispersion. It can be demonstrated that the ratio

$$(\text{the chi-square value})/(\text{degrees of freedom}) > 1$$

indicates the presence of over-dispersion, and

$$(\text{the chi-square value})/(\text{degrees of freedom}) \times \text{traditional se}$$

is an adequate adjustment for the over-dispersed se. The square root of this ratio is usually called the VIF (variance inflating factor).

4   Example of Making Your Own Assessment of Over-Dispersion

The underneath study assess the effect of beta-blockers and calcium channel blockers normalization of increased blood pressure in 831 patients. It uses a binary logistic model for analysis with normalization of blood pressure as outcome. Over-dispersion can be detected by goodness of fit tests. In the current example the Pearson's chi-square goodness of fit test is used. Because to data statistical software programs do not routinely account over-dispersion, investigators have to make their own assessments prior to the analysis.

Table 8.1 A hypothesized example of a 2 × 2 multi-centre factorial clinical trial of the effect of a beta-blocker and a calcium channel blocker on hypertension

Calcium channel blocker	Dummy calcium channel blocker							
	Dummy b-b		Beta-blocker		Dummy b-b		Beta-blocker	
Center	Resp	Total	Resp	Total	Resp	Total	Resp	Total
1	10	39	5	6	8	16	3	12
2	23	62	53	74	10	30	22	41
3	23	81	55	72	8	28	15	30
3	26	51	32	51	23	45	32	51
4	17	39	46	79	0	4	3	7
5			10	13				
Mean proportion per treatment combination								
	0.364		0.681		0.249		0.532	

b-b = beta-blocker
Resp = number of responders (a mean blood pressure under 107 mmHg)
Total = total number of patients with specific treatment combination per centre

Table 8.1 shows a hypothesized example of a 2 × 2 multi-centre factorial clinical trial of the effect of a beta-blocker and a calcium channel blocker on hypertension. The analysis requires the binary logistic model (ln = natural logarithm):

ln odds of responding = $a + b_1 x_1 + b_2 x_2 + b_3 x_1 x_2$
x_1 = beta-blocker
x_2 = calcium channel blocker

There is a strong difference in the total numbers of observations per centre: between 4 and 81. This could lead to over-dispersion. The Pearson goodness of fit test can be used to assess the presence of it. The calculation is given in Table 8.2. If we add up the other three treatment combination results to 10.0, we will end up with a chi-square value of 10.0 + ... = 32. This chi-square value should be approximately equal to its degrees of freedom for the logistic model to hold. We have, however, 21 (cells) – 4 (treatment combinations) = 17 degrees of freedom. This would mean that the data are over-dispersed. A solution recommended by Hojsgaard and Halekoh is used [8]. The magnitude of the dispersion can be estimated by the ratio:

chi-square number/degrees of freedom = 32/17 = 1.9

The square root of this ratio (here $\sqrt{1.9}$), sometimes called the variance inflating factor can, subsequently, be used to adjust the standard errors in the study. ln odds of responding = $a + b_1 x_1 + b_2 x_2 + b_3 x_1 x_2$ (ln = natural logarithm). The calculation is given in Table 8.3.

The probability of responding to a dummy beta-blocker and calcium channel blocker equals 0.36. This is unchanged after adjustment for dispersion. however, the 95 % confidence of this probability changes from 0.31–0.42 to 0.28–0.45. In conclusion, with over-dispersion the parameter estimates are not affected, but their standard errors are likely to be underestimated, and should be adjusted for that flaw.

Table 8.2 The Pearson goodness of fit test of the data of Table 1

$$\text{chi-square} = \sum \frac{(\text{observed numbers responders} - \text{expected numbers responders})^2}{\text{expected numbers responders}}$$

The calculation per treatment combination per centre is as follows

1. $(10 - 39 \times 0.364)/39 \times (10/39 - (1 - 10/39))$	$= 2.2$
2.	$= 0.0$
3.	$= 2.2$
4.	$= 4.5$
5.	$= 1.1 \quad +$
	$= 10.0$

Table 8.3 The calculation of a standard error adjusted for over-dispersion

		SE	p	SE_{adjust}	p
a	−0.41	0.18	0.025	0.25	0.119
b_1	0.54	0.25	0.031	0.34	0.132
b_2	−0.15	0.22	0.513	0.30	0.638
b_3	0.78	0.31	0.011	0.42	0.080

$SE_{adjust} = $ SE adjusted for over-dispersion $= \sqrt{1.9} \times SE$

5   Example of Using SPSS [6] for Assessing Over-Dispersion

The underneath example uses a Poisson regression for data analysis.

The primary questions were, do psychological and social factors affect the rates of episodes of torsades de pointes, are certain treatments efficacious in preventing the rates of torsades de pointes. Poisson regression is different from linear en logistic regression [9], because it uses a log transformed counts (here numbers of torsades de pointes) as dependent variable. For counts per time per group, otherwise called rates, defined as numbers of events per person per time unit, Poisson regression is very sensitive and probably better than standard regression methods. Fifty patients were followed for numbers of episodes of torsades de pointes, while on treated with two parallel treatment modalities. The data file is below. It is entitled "chap8over-dispersion.sav", and is electronically available on the internet at extras/springer.com.

Var 1	var 2	var 3	var 4 (var = variable)
1	56,99	42,45	4
1	37,09	46,82	4
0	32,28	43,57	2
0	29,06	43,57	3
0	6,75	27,25	3
0	61,65	48,41	13
0	56,99	40,74	11
1	10,39	15,36	7
1	50,53	52,12	10

(continued)

(continued)

1	49,47	42,45	9
0	39,56	36,45	4
1	33,74	13,13	5
0	62,91	62,27	5
0	65,56	44,66	3
1	23,01	25,25	1
1	75,83	61,04	0
0	41,31	49,47	1
0	41,89	65,56	0
1	65,56	46,82	2
1	13,13	6,75	24
0	33,02	42,45	2
1	55,88	64,87	0
1	45,21	55,34	1
1	56,99	44,66	0
0	31,51	38,35	8
1	52,65	50,00	3
1	17,26	6,75	7
0	33,02	40,15	0
1	61,04	57,55	2
1	66,98	71,83	0
1	1,01	45,21	0
0	38,35	35,13	1
1	44,66	46,82	3
1	44,12	46,82	0
1	59,85	46,29	0
0	32,28	47,35	28
1	23,01	49,47	8
1	70,94	61,04	5
1	1,01	1,01	2
0	41,89	52,12	27
0	40,15	35,13	5
0	41,31	38,35	18
0	44,66	58,69	19
1	38,35	42,45	9
1	32,28	1,01	9
0	37,09	32,28	4
1	63,55	57,55	2
1	43,57	41,31	3
1	33,02	24,17	9
0	68,49	59,26	20

Var 1 = treatment modality; var 2 = psychological score; var 3 = social score; var 5 = numbers of episodes of torsades de pointe

First, we will perform a linear regression analysis with var 4 as outcome variable and the other 3 variables as predictors.

Command: Analyze….Regression….Linear….Dependent Variable: episodes of torsades de pointes….Independent: treatment modality, psychological score, social score….OK.

Table 8.4 Multiple linear regression with torsades de pointes as outcome and three predictor variables

Coefficients[a]

Model	Unstandardized coefficients		Standardized coefficients		
	B	Std. error	Beta	t	Sig.
1 (Constant)	11,271	3,163		3,563	,001
treatment modality	−4,373	2,039	−,306	−2,144	,037
psychological score	,021	,077	,055	,277	,783
social score	−,083	,086	−,193	−,974	,335

[a]Dependent Variable: torsades de pointes

Table 8.5 Multiple Poisson regression with the chance of torsades de pointes as outcome

Parameter estimates

Parameter	B	Std. error	95 % Wald confidence interval		Hypothesis test		
			Lower	Upper	Wald chi-square	df	Sig.
(Intercept)	1,921	,1658	1,597	2,246	134,364	1	,000
[treat = 0]	,736	,1217	,497	,974	36,571	1	,000
[treat = 1]	0[a]	.	.	.	.	.	.
psych	,004	,0046	,005	,013	,638	1	,425
soc	−,015	,0052	−,026	−,005	8.822	1	,003
(Scale)	1[b]						

Dependent variable: torsades de pointes
Model: (Intercept), treat, psych, soc
[a]Set to Zero because this parameter is redundant
[b]Fixed at the displayed value

Table 8.4 shows that treatment modality is weakly significant, and psychological and social score are not. For rate values Poisson regression with the log rate (numbers of torsades de pointes) as dependent variable may be a more sensitive method than linear regression.

Command: Generalized Linear Models....mark: Custom....Distribution: Poisson..... Link function: Log.... Response: Dependent variable: numbers of episodes of torsades de pointes....Scale Weight Variable: days of observation....Predictors: Main Effect: treatment modality....Covariates: psychological score, social score.... Model: main effects: treatment modality, psychological score, social score.... Estimation: mark Model- based Estimation....OK.

Table 8.5 gives the results. Both the treatment modality and the social score are now significant predictors of the chance of torsades de pointes. The output sheets also give a table of goodness of fit tests (Table 8.6). The Deviance and Pearson chi-square values are 6.764 and 7,259. These values should be near 1. The fact that they are (much) greater, indicate that an over-dispersed model is probable. A formal test to determine whether there is over-dispersion is a so-called negative binomial with log link as model. Table 8.7 gives the goodness of fit tests. The log likelihood value is larger, −227.001 and −140.459 respectively. Also the Deviance and Pearson

Table 8.6 Goodness of fit tests of the Poisson regression model with log torsades de pointes as dependent variable

Goodness of fit[b]

	Value	df	Value/df
Deviance	311,143	46	6,764
Scaled Deviance	311,143	46	
Pearson Chi-Square	333,919	46	7,259
Scaled Pearson Chi-Square	333,919	46	
Log Likelihood[a]	−227,001		
Akaike's Information Criterion (AIC)	462,001		
Finite Sample Corrected AIC (AICC)	462,890		
Bayesian Information Criterion (BIC)	469,649		
Consistent AIC (CAIC)	473,649		

Dependent variable: torsades de pointes
Model: (Intercept), treat, psych, soc
[a]The full log likelihood function is displayed and used in computing information criteria
[b]Information criteria are in small-is-better form

Table 8.7 Goodness of fit tests of the negative binomial with log link model, log torsades de pointes is again the dependent variable

Goodness of fit[b]

	Value	df	Value/df
Deviance	57,323	46	1,246
Scaled Deviance	57,323	46	
Pearson Chi-Square	44,498	46	,967
Scaled Pearson Chi-Square	44,498	46	
Log Likelihood[a]	−140,459		
Akaike's Information Criterion (AIC)	288,917		
Finite Sample Corrected AIC (AICC)	289,806		
Bayesian Information Criterion (BIC)	296,565		
Consistent AIC (CAIC)	300,565		

Dependent variable: torsades de pointes
Model: (Intercept), treat, psych, soc
[a]The full log likelihood function is displayed and used in computing information criteria
[b]Information criteria are in small-is-better form

chi-square values are much smaller, 1.246 and 0.967, both of them close to 1.0. This would mean that the effect of over-dispersion has been removed by this model.

Table 8.8 finally shows that the Poisson model adjusted for over-dispersion provides larger Wald-values and p-values. The p-value for treatment modality rose from 0.0001 to 0.007. The p-value for social score from 0.003 to 0.164. According to this model the psychological and social scores are not significant predictors of the chance of torsades de pointes. This was in agreement with the investigators' prior hypothesis that these factors are kind of placebo effects rather than true effects.

Table 8.8 Poisson regression with the negative binomial with log link model

Parameter estimates

Parameter	B	Std. error	95 % Wald confidence interval Lower	Upper	Hypothesis test Wald chi-square	df	Sig.
(Intercept)	2,089	,4389	1,229	2,949	22,654	1	,000
[treat = 0]	,906	,3357	,249	1,564	7,293	1	,007
[treat = 1]	0[a]	.	.	.	.	.	.
psych	,002	,0134	−,025	,028	,015	1	,902
soc	−,020	,0140	−,047	,008	1,933	1	,164
(Scale)	1[b]						
(Negative binomial)	1						

Dependent variable: torsades de pointes
Model: (Intercept), treat, psych, soc
[a]Set to Zero because this parameter is redundant
[b]Fixed at the displayed value

6 Discussion

Binary datasets are particularly at risk of over-dispersion, because their variance is underestimated by traditional methods, due to dependencies between binary sequences, but any other type of data may involve over-dispersion [1–5]. Conclusions from traditional analyses of data with over-dispersion should be interpreted with caution, because the calculated confidence intervals and p-values are too small and the conclusion of a significant effect may erroneously be made [1–5]. Particularly, if a strong difference in numbers of responders or magnitudes of responses is in the data, the presence of over-dispersion should be assessed. Goodness of fit tests are available for that purpose. The advantage of the Pearson chi-square goodness of fit test, is, that, in addition to detecting over-dispersion, it enables to adjust for it [8]. The adjusted mean of the data remains unchanged, while the measures of dispersion in the data, including variances and co-variances, log – likelihoods, Wald – intervals etc. are, simply, multiplied by the square root of the ratio of the chi-square value and its degrees of freedom (variance inflating factor = chi-square/degrees of freedom). Although assessment of over-dispersion is not yet widely applied, SPSS [6] offers the possibility to assess binary data with a Poisson regression model largely adjusted for over-dispersion. We recommend that analytical methods in clinical research should always try and include a measure of dispersion in the data. With large differences in the data, the presence of over-dispersion should be assessed and adjusted.

7 Conclusions

1. Over-dispersion means that the spread in the data is wider than compatible with Gaussian modeling. Traditional statistical tests overestimate the precision of over-dispersed data, meaning that the calculated p-values are too small, and the conclusion of a significant effect is erroneously made.
2. Over-dispersion is more commonly observed with binary data than it is with continuous data.
3. Several tests are available but Pearson goodness of fit test is often used to assess and adjust over-dispersion.
4. For binary data SPSS offers a Poisson model adjusted for over-dispersion.
5. With large differences in the data, the presence of over-dispersion should be assessed and adjusted.
6. Non-mathematicians are able to do so either with or without the help of SPSS tests especially developed for the purpose.

References

1. Anonymous (2013) Overdispersion. At Planet Math. http://planetmath.org/encyclopedia/Overdispersion.html. 26 June 2013
2. Cleophas TJ, Zwinderman AH (2012) Data dispersion issues. In: Cleophas TJ, Zwinderman AH (eds) Statistics applied to clinical studies, 5th edn. Springer, Heidelberg, pp 149–159
3. Fisher R (1953) Dispersion on a sphere. Proc R Soc Lond 217:295–305
4. Tan M (2003) Describing data, variability, and overdispersion in medical research. In: Fang J (ed) Advanced medical statistics. World Scientific, River Edge, pp 319–332
5. Hojsgaard S, Halekoh U (2005) Overdispersion. Danish Institute of Agricultural Sciences, Copenhagen, 1 June. http://gbi.agrsci.dk/statistics/courses. 26 June 2013
6. SPSS Statistical Software (2013) www.spss.com. 26 June 2013
7. Anonymous (2013) Gauss summary. www-groups.dcs.st-and.ac.uk/history/Mathematicians/Gauss.html. 26 June 2013
8. Cleophas TJ, Zwinderman AH (2012) Testing clinical trials for randomness. In: Cleophas TJ, Zwinderman AH (eds) Statistics applied to clinical studies, 5th edn. Springer, Heidelberg, pp 469–478
9. Cleophas TJ, Zwinderman AH (2012) Poisson regression. In: Cleophas TJ, Zwinderman AH (eds) SPSS for starters part two. Springer, Heidelberg, pp 43–48

Chapter 9
Random Effects

1 Summary

1.1 Background

In clinical trials it is common to assume a fixed effects research model. This means that the patients are homogeneous and differences observed are residual, i.e. due to chance. If certain patients due to co-morbidity, co-medication, age or other factors will respond differently from others, then the spread in the data is caused not only by the residual effect but also by subgroup properties.

1.2 Objective

To assess random effects modeling as an appropriate methodology for hidden and unexpected subgroup properties.

1.3 Methods

Two real data studies were used as examples, (1) one with interaction between gender and treatment modality, (2) one with a positive correlation between repeated measures in one subject. SPSS's modules General linear model and Mixed linear modeling were used for random effects analyses.

T.J. Cleophas and A.H. Zwinderman, *Machine Learning in Medicine: Part Three*,
DOI 10.1007/978-94-007-7869-6_9, © Springer Science+Business Media Dordrecht 2013

1.4   Results

The random effects analyses showed that (1) the overall p-values were, rightly, no longer significant, and that (2) instead of insignificant very significant treatment effects were obtained.

1.5   Conclusions

1. In clinical trials a fixed effects research model assumes that the patients selected for a specific treatment have the same true quantitative effect and that the differences observed are residual error. If, however, we have reasons to believe that certain patients respond differently from others, then the spread in the data is caused not only by the residual error but also by between patient differences. The latter situation requires a random effects model.
2. In studies with a significant interaction between treatment effect and some subgroup effect, an overall data analysis is rather meaningless, and a random effects analysis should be performed. It is available in SPSS.
3. Studies with repeated measurements should be account the correlation between the repeated measures in one subject. Random effects analysis using the mixed linear module in SPSS is appropriate for the purpose.
4. Random effects research models enable the assessment of an entire sample of data for subgroup differences without need to split the data into subgroups.
5. Clinical investigators are generally hardly aware of this possibility and, therefore, wrongly assess random effects as fixed effects leading to a biased interpretation of the data.

2   Introduction

In clinical trials it is common to assume a fixed effects research model. This means that the patients selected for a specific treatment are assumed to be homogeneous and have the same true quantitative effect and that the differences observed are residual, meaning that they are caused by inherent variability in biological processes, rather than some hidden subgroup property. If, however, we have reasons to believe that certain patients due to co-morbidity, co-medication, age or other factors will respond differently from others, then the spread in the data is caused not only by the residual effect but also by between patient differences due to some subgroup property. It may even be safe to routinely treat any patient effect as a random effect, unless there are good arguments no to do so. Random effects research models require a statistical approach different from that of fixed effects

Models [1–3]. With the fixed effects model the treatment differences are tested against the residual error, otherwise called the standard error. With the random effects models the treatment effects may be influenced not only by the residual effect but also by some unexpected, otherwise called random, factor, and so the treatment should no longer be tested against the residual effect. Because both residual and random effect constitute a much larger amount of uncertainty in the data, the treatment effect has to be tested against both of them [4, 5].

Random effects models have been used in several studies recently published [6–12]. They are a very interesting class of models, but even a partial understanding is fairly difficult to achieve. This chapter was written to explain random effects models in analysis of variance and to give examples of studies qualifying for them.

Real data examples are given. Step-by-step analyses are performed.

3 Example 1, a Parallel Group Trial with Gender as Random Effect (Table 9.1)

A 40 patient parallel group study of the effects of metoprolol and verapamil on numbers of paroxysmal atrial tachycardia (PAT) episodes is studied. The primary scientific question: is there interaction between the effects of gender and treatment on the treatment outcome.

Overall, metoprolol seems to perform better. However, this is only true only for one subgroup (males). The presence of interaction between gender and treatment modality can be assessed several ways: (1) t-tests [13], (2) analysis of variance, and (3) regression analysis. The data file is in Table 9.2. It is entitled "chap9random1.sav", and can be downloaded from the internet at extra.springer.com.

We will first perform an analysis of variance using SPSS statistical software [14].

Command: Analyze….General linear model….Univariate analysis of variance ….Dependent variable:episode PAT….Fixed factors:treatment, gender….OK

Table 9.3 shows that there is a significant interaction between gender and treatment at $p = 0.0001$ (var 2* var 3, * is sign of multiplication). In spite of this the treatment modality is a significant predictor of the outcome. In situations like this it is often better to use a *random* effect model. The sum of squares treatment is then compared to the sum of squares interaction instead of the sum of squares error. This is a good idea since the interaction was unexpected, and is a major contributor to the error, otherwise called spread, in the data. This would mean that we have much more spread in the data than expected and we will lose a lot of power to prove whether or not the treatment is a significant predictor of the outcome, episodes of PAT. Random effect analysis of variance requires the following commands:

Command: Analyze….General linear model….Univariate analysis of variance …. Dependent Variable: episodes of PAT….Fixed Factors: treatment…. Random Factors: gender….OK.

Table 9.1 Data of Example 1

Verapamil	Metoprolol	
Males		
52	28	
48	35	
43	34	
50	32	
43	34	
44	27	
46	31	
46	27	
43	29	
49+	25+	
464	302	766
Females		
38	43	
42	34	
42	33	
35	42	
33	41	
38	37	
39	37	
34	40	
33	36	
34+	35+	
368	378	746
832	680	

Table 9.4 shows the results. As expected the interaction effect remained statistically significant, but the treatment effect has now lost its significance. This is realistic, since in a trial with major interactions, an overall treatment effect analysis is not relevant anymore. A better approach will be a separate analysis of the treatment effect in the subgroups that caused the interaction.

As a contrast test we will also use regression analysis for these data. For that purpose we first have to add an interaction variable: interaction variable = treatment modality * gender (* = sign of multiplication). The previously given data file shows the calculated interaction variable in the 4th column. The interaction variable is then used together with treatment modality and gender as independent variables in a multiple linear regression model.

Command: Analyze....Regression....Linear....Dependent: episodes PAT ....Independent: treatment modality, gender, interaction....OK.

Table 9.5 shows the results of the multiple linear regression. Like with fixed effect analysis of variance, both treatment modality and interaction are statistically significant. The t-value-interaction of the regression = 7.932. The F-value-interaction of the fixed effect analysis of variance = 62.916 and this equals 7.932^2.

Table 9.2 SPSS data file of Example 1

Var 1	Var 2	Var 3	Var 4 (var = variable)
52,00	0,00	0,00	0,00
48,00	0,00	0,00	0,00
43,00	0,00	0,00	0,00
50,00	0,00	0,00	0,00
43,00	0,00	0,00	0,00
44,00	0,00	0,00	0,00
46,00	0,00	0,00	0,00
46,00	0,00	0,00	0,00
43,00	0,00	0,00	0,00
49,00	0,00	0,00	0,00
28,00	1,00	0,00	0,00
35,00	1,00	0,00	0,00
34,00	1,00	0,00	0,00
32,00	1,00	0,00	0,00
34,00	1,00	0,00	0,00
27,00	1,00	0,00	0,00
31,00	1,00	0,00	0,00
27,00	1,00	0,00	0,00
29,00	1,00	0,00	0,00
25,00	1,00	0,00	0,00
38,00	0,00	1,00	0,00
42,00	0,00	1,00	0,00
42,00	0,00	1,00	0,00
35,00	0,00	1,00	0,00
33,00	0,00	1,00	0,00
38,00	0,00	1,00	0,00
39,00	0,00	1,00	0,00
34,00	0,00	1,00	0,00
33,00	0,00	1,00	0,00
34,00	0,00	1,00	0,00
43,00	1,00	1,00	1,00
34,00	1,00	1,00	1,00
33,00	1,00	1,00	1,00
42,00	1,00	1,00	1,00
41,00	1,00	1,00	1,00
37,00	1,00	1,00	1,00
37,00	1,00	1,00	1,00
40,00	1,00	1,00	1,00
36,00	1,00	1,00	1,00
35,00	1,00	1,00	1,00

Var 1 = number of episodes of paroxysmal atrial tachycardia (PAT)
Var 2 = treatment modality (0 = verapamil, 1 = metoprolol)
Var 3 = gender (0 = male, 1 = female)
Var 4 = interaction variable = treatment modality*gender
(* = sign of multiplication)

Table 9.3 Fixed effects analysis of variance of Example 1 showing a significant interaction between gender (Var 3) and treatment (Var 2)

Tests of between-subjects effects

Dependent variable:epsiodes PAF

Source	Type III sum of squares	df	Mean square	F	Sig.
Corrected model	1327,200[a]	3	442,400	37,633	,000
Intercept	57153,600	1	57153,600	4861,837	,000
VAR00002	577,600	1	577,600	49,134	,000
VAR00003	10,000	1	10,000	,851	,363
VAR00002* VAR00003	739,600	1	739,600	62,915	,000
Error	423,200	36	11,756		
Total	58904,000	40			
Corrected total	1750,400	39			

[a]R squared = ,758 (adjusted R squared = ,738)

Table 9.4 Random effects analysis of variance of Example 1 showing a significant interaction between gender (Var 3) and treatment (Var 2), and insignificant effects of treatment (Var 2) and gender (Var 3)

Tests of between-subjects effects

Dependent variable:VAR00001

Source		Type III sum of squares	df	Mean square	F	Sig.
Intercept	Hypothesis	57153,600	1	57153,600	98,950	,064
	Error	577,600	1	577,600[a]		
VAR00003	Hypothesis	10,000	1	10,000	,014	,926
	Error	739,600	1	739,600[b]		
VAR00002	Hypothesis	577,600	1	577,600	,781	.539
	Error	739,600	1	739,600[b]		
VAR00003 * VAR00002	Hypothesis	739,600	1	739,600	62,915	,000
	Error	423,200	36	11,756[c]		

[a]MS(VAR00002)
[b]MS(VAR00003 * VAR00002)
[c]MS(Error)

Table 9.5 Fixed effects multiple linear regression with numbers of PAT as outcome variable

Coefficients[a]

Model		Unstandardized coefficients		Standardized coefficients		
		B	Std. error	Beta	t	Sig.
1	(Constant)	46,400	1,084		42,795	,000
	treatment	−16,200	1,533	−1,224	−10,565	,000
	gender	−9,600	1,533	−,726	−6,261	,000
	interaction	17,200	2,168	1,126	7,932	,000

[a]Dependent variable: outcome

Obviously, the two approaches make use of a very similar arithmetic. Unfortunately, for random effect regression SPSS has limited possibilities.

4 Example 2, a Parallel Group Study with a Positive Correlation Between Repeated Measurements as Random Effect

A parallel group study with a positive correlation between repeated measurements as random effect. The data file are in Table 9.6. It is entitled "chap9random2.sav", and can be downloaded from the internet at extra.springer.com. It is appropriate, whenever possible, to use a summary estimate of repeated data. For example, the area under the curve of drug concentration-time curves is used in clinical pharmacology as an estimate of bioavailability of a drug. Also, maximal values, mean values, changes from baseline are applied for the same purpose. The disadvantage of this approach is, that it does not use the data fully, because summary measures are used instead of the individual data, and, therefore, precision may be lost, but, otherwise, the approach is unbiased, and can be used perfectly well. As an alternative and more precise method a mixed-linear model, as reviewed below, using the covariance between the repeated measures as a random effect, can be used.

| Table 9.6 Original data file | HDL cholesterol measurements | | | | | |
of twenty patient parallel group study of two treatments for HDL cholesterol: patients are measured once in 5 subsequent weeks	Pat no	1st	2nd	3rd	4th	5th	Treatment modality
	1	1,66	1,62	1,57	1,52	1,50	0,00
	2	1,69	1,71	1,60	1,55	1,56	0,00
	3	1,92	1,94	1,83	1,78	1,79	0,00
	4	1,95	1,97	1,86	1,81	1,82	0,00
	5	1,98	2,00	1,89	1,84	1,85	0,00
	6	2,01	2,03	1,92	1,87	1,88	0,00
	7	2,04	2,06	1,95	1,90	1,91	0,00
	8	2,07	2,09	1,98	1,93	1,94	0,00
	9	2,30	2,32	2,21	2,16	2,17	0,00
	10	2,36	2,35	2,26	2,23	2,20	0,00
	11	1,57	1,82	1,83	1,83	1,82	1,00
	12	1,60	1,85	1,89	1,89	1,85	1,00
	13	1,83	2,08	2,12	2,12	2,08	1,00
	14	1,86	2,11	2,16	2,15	2,11	1,00
	15	2,80	2,14	2,19	2,18	2,14	1,00
	16	1,92	2,17	2,22	2,21	2,17	1,00
	17	1,95	2,20	2,25	2,24	2,20	1,00
	18	1,98	2,23	2,28	2,27	2,24	1,00
	19	2,21	2,46	2,57	2,51	2,48	1,00
	20	2,34	2,51	2,55	2,55	2,52	1,00

In the example is given of a parallel group study of the effect of two statins on HDL cholesterol. HDL cholesterol is measured every week for 5 weeks. The averages of the 5 repeated measures in one patient are calculated and an unpaired t-test was used to compare these averages in the two treatment groups. The overall average in group 0 was 1.925 (SEM 0.0025), in group 1 2.227 (SE 0.227). With 18 degrees of freedom and a t-value of 1.99 the difference did not obtain statistical significance, $0.05 < p < 0.10$. There seems to be, expectedly, a strong positive correlation between the 5 repeated measurements in one patient. In order to take account of this strong positive correlation a random-effects mixed-linear model is used. For this particular analysis all measurements have to be ordered in a single column, not in 5 columns side by side. In a second column the time of the separate measurements have to be noted. SPSS statistical software is used for the analysis. Before a mixed linear analysis can be executed, first the data file has to be restructured. Restructuring will be performed using SPSS (Table 9.7).[14]

Command: Data....Restructure....click Restructure Selected Variables....Step 2 of 7.... select One....Step 3 of 7....select Case number as identity....select 1st to 5th cholesterol measurement to be transported....Step 3 of 7.....select treatment as 2nd target variable.... Step 4 of 7 select One....Step 5 of 7....type time as variable label....click Finish.

The restructured data file will now be used for both a fixed and a random effects analysis using the module mixed linear modeling in SPSS.[14]

Command: Mixed Model....Linear....Subjects: enter case....Repeated: enter Time.... click Continue....Dependent: enter HDL cholesterol....Factor: enter Time....click Fixed....select Time in Factors and Covariates box....click Add....click Statistics....select Parameter estimates....click Continue....click OK..

In the output sheets the statistics of the fixed effect model is given (Table 9.8). The test statistics are large: the smaller the better. If a fixed model is used, at none of the times 1–5 the treatment modality is a significant predictor of the HDL cholesterol at that time (Table 9.9). A random effects analysis will be, subsequently, performed.

Command: Mixed Model....Linear....Subjects: enter case....Repeated:Time....Repeated Covariance-Type: select Unstructured....click Continue....Dependent: enter HDL cholesterol....Factor: enter Time....click Fixed....select Time in Factors and Covariates box....click Add....click Statistics....select Parameter estimates....click Continue.... click OK..

The output sheets show that the test statistics are now very small (Table 9.10). This is good. The random effects model shows that at virtually all of the times the treatment modality is a significant predictor of the HDL cholesterol levels (Table 9.11). It can be observed that the overall mean cholesterol in the two analyses is equal: 2.011500 (the Intercept of the mixed linear model). Also the differences from the mean are similar. However, their standard errors are largely different.

Table 9.7 Restructured data from Table 9.6

Pat no	Treat modal	Time (week)	HDL cholesterol
1	0,00	1	1,66
1	0,00	2	1,62
1	0,00	3	1,57
1	0,00	4	1,52
1	0,00	5	1,50
2	0,00	1	1,69
2	0,00	2	1,71
2	0,00	3	1,60
2	0,00	4	1,55
2	0,00	5	1,56
3	0,00	1	1,92
3	0,00	2	1,94
3	0,00	3	1,83
3	0,00	4	1,78
3	0,00	5	1,79
4	0,00	1	1,95
4	0,00	2	1,97
4	0,00	3	1,86
4	0,00	4	1,81
4	0,00	5	1,82
5	0,00	1	1,98
5	0,00	2	2,00
5	0,00	3	1,89
5	0,00	4	1,84
5	0,00	5	1,85
6	0,00	1	2,01
6	0,00	2	2,03
6	0,00	3	1,92
6	0,00	4	1,87
6	0,00	5	1,88
7	0,00	1	2,04
7	0,00	2	2,06
7	0,00	3	1,95
7	0,00	4	1,90
7	0,00	5	1,91
8	0,00	1	2,07
8	0,00	2	2,09
8	0,00	3	1,98
8	0,00	4	1,93
8	0,00	5	1,94
9	0,00	1	2,30
9	0,00	2	2,32
9	0,00	3	2,21
9	0,00	4	2,16
9	0,00	5	2,17
10	0,00	1	2,36
10	0,00	2	2,35
10	0,00	3	2,26
10	0,00	4	2,23
10	0,00	5	2,20

(continued)

Table 9.7 (continued)

Pat no	Treat modal	Time (week)	HDL cholesterol
11	1,00	1	1,57
11	1,00	2	1,82
11	1,00	3	1,83
11	1,00	4	1,83
11	1,00	5	1,82
12	1,00	1	1,60
12	1,00	2	1,85
12	1,00	3	1,89
12	1,00	4	1,89
12	1,00	5	1,85
13	1,00	1	1,83
13	1,00	2	2,08
13	1,00	3	2,12
13	1,00	4	2,12
13	1,00	5	2,08
14	1,00	1	1,86
14	1,00	2	2,11
14	1,00	3	2,16
14	1,00	4	2,15
14	1,00	5	2,11
15	1,00	1	2,80
15	1,00	2	2,14
15	1,00	3	2,19
15	1,00	4	2,18
15	1,00	5	2,14
16	1,00	1	1,92
16	1,00	2	2,17
16	1,00	3	2,22
16	1,00	4	2,21
16	1,00	5	2,17
17	1,00	1	1,95
17	1,00	2	2,20
17	1,00	3	2,25
17	1,00	4	2,24
17	1,00	5	2,20
18	1,00	1	1,98
18	1,00	2	2,23
18	1,00	3	2,28
18	1,00	4	2,27
18	1,00	5	2,24
19	1,00	1	2,21
19	1,00	2	2,46
19	1,00	3	2,57
19	1,00	4	2,51
19	1,00	5	2,48
20	1,00	1	2,34
20	1,00	2	2,51
20	1,00	3	2,55
20	1,00	4	2,55
20	1,00	5	2,52

Table 9.8 The statistics of the fixed effects analysis using the mixed linear module in SPSS

Information criteria[a]	
−2 Restricted Log Likelihood	34,375
Akaike's Information Criterion (AIC)	44,375
Hurvich and Tsai's Criterion (AICC)	45,049
Bozdogan's Criterion (CAIC)	62,145
Schwarz's Bayesian Criterian (BIC)	57,145

The information criteria are displayed in smaller-is-better forms
[a]Dependent variable: HDL cholesterol

Table 9.9 Mean results and their spread during 1st to 5th HDL cholesterol measurement (after 1–5 weeks treatment)

Estimates of fixed effects[b]

Parameter	Estimate	Std. error	df	t	Sig.	95 % confidence interval	
						Lower bound	Upper bound
Intercept	2,011500	,059720	19	33,682	,000	1,886505	2,136495
[time = 1]	−,009500	,088923	37,639	−,107	,915	−,189572	,170572
[time = 2]	,071500	,079048	37,254	,905	,372	−,088630	,231630
[time = 3]	,045000	,085096	37,991	,529	,600	−,127269	,217269
[time = 4]	,015500	,086473	37,919	,179	,859	−,159567	,190567
[time = 5]	0[a]	0	.	.	.	.	.

[a]This parameter is set to zero because it is redundant
[b]Dependent variable: HDL cholesterol

Table 9.10 The statistics of the random effects analysis using the mixed linear module in SPSS

Information criteria[a]	
−2 Restricted Log Likelihood	−265,644
Akaike's Information Criterion (AIC)	−235,644
Hurvich and Tsai's Criterion (AICC)	−229,569
Bozdogan's Criterion (CAIC)	−182,336
Schwarz's Bayesian Criterian (BIC)	−197,336

The information criteria are displayed in smaller-is-better forms
[a]Dependent variable: HDL cholesterol

Table 9.11 Mean results and their spread during 1st to 5th HDL cholesterol measurement (After 1–5 weeks treatment) using a random effects model

Estimates of fixed effects[b]

Parameter	Estimate	Std. error	df	t	Sig.	95 % confidence interval	
						Lower bound	Upper bound
Intercept	2,011500	,59720	19,001	33,682	,000	1,886505	2,136495
[time = 1]	−,009500	,055443	19,000	−,171	,866	−,125544	,106544
[time = 2]	,071500	,017416	19,000	4,106	,001	,035049	,107951
[time = 3]	,045000	,003517	19,000	12,795	,000	,037639	,052361
[time = 4]	,015500	,005051	19,000	3,069	,006	,004928	,026072
[time = 5]	0[a]	0	.	.	.	.	.

[a]This parameter is set to zero because it is redundant
[b]Dependent variable: HDL cholesterol

5   Discussion

In this chapter research models are discussed that account for variables with random rather than fixed effects. These models are often called type 2 models if they include random exposure variables and type 3 models if they include both fixed and random exposure variables. Both the examples 1 and 2 in this chapter gives a type 3 models, otherwise called mixed effects models.

The work-up of these advanced research models is sometimes largely the same as that of simple research models. But, inferences made are quite different. All inferences made under the simple model mostly concern means and differences between means. In contrast, the inferences made using advanced models deal with variances, and involve small differences between subsets of patients or between individual patients. This type of analysis of variance answers questions like: do differences between assessors, between classrooms, between institutions, or between subjects contribute to the overall variability in the data?

We should consider some limitations of the methods. If the experimenter chooses the wrong model, he/she may suffer from a loss of power. Also the standards of homogeneity / heterogeneity in the data must be taken seriously. The patients in the subsets should not be sort of alike, rather they should be exactly alike on the variable to be assessed. Often this assumption can not be adequately met, raising the risk of a biased interpretation of the data.

The random effects research models enable to assess the entire sample for the presence of possible differences between subgroups without need to, actually, split the data into subgroups. This very point is a major argument in their favor. Also they are, of course, more appropriate if variables can be assumed to be random rather than fixed. A potential disadvantage is that the sensitivity to detect a significant difference in the data is sometimes somewhat reduced. This is, because they are more complex and account more, and are therefore, sometimes, less sensitive than simple methods. However, if the model fits the data well, sensitivity may be rather improved as shown in the random effects analysis of example 2 in this chapter.

Also, the reduction of sensitivity should not be regarded as a disadvantage, but rather an advantage, since the chance to make a correct conclusion is increased. Data should be analyzed according to the correct procedure, not according to the procedure that gives the largest chance to demonstrate a significant difference.

Only the simplest examples have been given in the present paper. The Internet provides an overwhelming body of information on the advanced research models including the type 2 and 3 research models as discussed here. E.g., the Google data system provides 495,000 references for explanatory texts on this subject. This illustrates the enormous attention currently given to these upcoming techniques. Yet in clinical research these models are little known. We hope that this chapter will stimulate clinical investigators to more often apply them.

6 Conclusions

1. In clinical trials a fixed effects research model assumes that the patients selected for a specific treatment have the same true quantitative effect and that the differences observed are residual error. If, however, we have reasons to believe that certain patients respond differently from others, then the spread in the data is caused not only by the residual error but also by between patient differences. The latter situation requires a random effects model.
2. In studies with a significant interaction between treatment effect and some subgroup effect, an overall data analysis is rather meaningless, and a random effects analysis should be performed. It is available in SPSS [14].
3. Studies with repeated measurements should be account the correlation between the repeated measures in one subject. Random effects analysis using the mixed linear module in SPSS is appropriate for the purpose.
4. Random effects research models enable the assessment of an entire sample of data for subgroup differences without need to split the data into subgroups.
5. Clinical investigators are generally hardly aware of this possibility and, therefore, wrongly assess random effects as fixed effects leading to a biased interpretation of the data.

References

1. Anonymous (2006) Distinguishing between random and fixed variables, effects and coefficients. Newson, USP 656 Winter 2006, pp 1–3
2. Campbell MJ (2006) Random effects models. In: Campbell MJ (ed) Statistics at square two, 2nd edn. Blackwell Publishing/BMJ Books, Oxford, pp 67–83
3. Gao S (2003) Special models for sampling survey. In: Lu Y, Fang J (eds) Advanced medical statistics, 1st edn. World Scientific, River Edge, pp 685–709
4. Anonymous (2013) Variance components and mixed models. http://www.statsoft.com/text book/stvarcom.html. 9 Feb 2013
5. Anonymous (2013) Random effects models. Wikipedia, the free encyclopedia. http://en. wikipedia.org/wiki/random-effects_models.html. 9 Feb 2013
6. Brier ME, Aronoff GR (1996) Application of artificial neural networks to clinical pharmacology. Int J Clin Pharmacol Ther 34:510–514
7. Dalla Costa T, Nolting A, Rand K, Derendorf H (1997) Pharmacokinetic -pharmacodynamic modelling of the in vitro antiinfective effect of piperacillin -tazobactam combinations. Int J Clin Pharmacol Ther 35:426–433
8. Mahmood I (2003) Center specificity in the limited sampling model (LSM): can the LSM developed from healthy subjects be extended to disease states? Int J Clin Pharmacol Ther 41:517–523
9. Meibohm B, Derendorf H (1997) Basic concepts of pharmacokinetic/pharmacodynamic (PK/PD) modelling. Int J Clin Pharmacol Ther 35:401–413
10. Lima JJ, Beasley BN, Parker RB, Johnson JA (2005) A pharmacodynamic model of the effects of controlled-onset extended-release verapamil on 24-hour ambulatory blood pressure. Int J Clin Pharmacol Ther 43:187–194
11. Lotsch J, Kobal G, Geisslinger G (2004) Programming of a flexible computer simulation to visualize pharmacokinetic-pharmacodynamic models. Int J Clin Pharmacol Ther 42:15–22

12. Mueck W, Becka M, Kubitza D, Voith B, Zuehlsdorf M (2007) Population model of the pharmacokinetics and pharmacodynamics of rivaroxaban–an oral, direct factor xa inhibitor–in healthy subjects. Int J Clin Pharmacol Ther 45:335–344

13. Cleophas TJ, Zwinderman AH (2011) Interaction, chapter 18. In: Cleophas TJ, Zwinderman AH (eds) Statistical analysis of clinical data on a pocket calculator. Springer, Heidelberg, pp 49–51

14. SPSS Statistical Software (2013) http://www.spss.com. 9 Feb 2013

Chapter 10
Weighted Least Squares

1 Summary

1.1 Background

Linear regression assumes that the spread of the outcome-values is the same for each predictor value. This assumption is, however, not warranted in many real life situations.

1.2 Objective

To assess the advantages of weighted least squares (WLS) instead of ordinary least squares (OLS) linear regression analysis.

1.3 Methods

A 78 patient simulated sample of the effect of different dosages of prednisone and beta agonist on peak expiratory flow in bronchial asthma was used.

1.4 Results

The WLS produced better statistics: the r value rose from 0.763 to 0.846, the t-values rose from 10 and 0.5 to 14 and 3.2. The p-values fell from 0.000 and 0.552 to respectively 0.000 and 0.002.

T.J. Cleophas and A.H. Zwinderman, *Machine Learning in Medicine: Part Three*, 95
DOI 10.1007/978-94-007-7869-6_10, © Springer Science+Business Media Dordrecht 2013

1.5   Conclusions

1. The current paper shows that, even with a sample of only 78 patients, WLS is able to demonstrate statistically significant linear effects that had been, previously, obscured by heteroscedasticity of the y-value.
2. The most precise regression estimates can be obtained by using weighted least squares linear regression with weights inversely proportional to the standard deviations as observed.
3. This is, however, an ideal situation. In practice, outlier standard deviations are usually applied for several values, and this carries the risk of overestimating the effects of the outliers.
4. Another disadvantage is that you use weights that you, actually, don't know or, at best, only know approximately.
5. A final disadvantage is the lack of power of the weights, particularly with small data. SPSS only accepts weighted variance solutions, if the power is >50 %, i.e., and the chance of a false negative result (or type II error) <50 %.
6. Weighted least squares is more precise in real life data than linear regression is.

2   Introduction

Linear regression assumes that the spread of the outcome-values is the same for each predictor value. This assumption is, however, not warranted in many real life situations. Particularly, it is often observed that the larger the predictor values, the more spread will observed in the outcome values. This, at the same time, means, that, with increasing predictor values, outcome errors rise, and that uncertainty will be inflated. Normally, with linear regression, the best fit regression equation is computed from the means of the squared distances from the data to the regression line. The regression line is the best fit line, no other line provides a smaller sum of squared distances. However, in the situation where the spread of the outcome values around the best regression line is not constant, the usual least sum of squares procedure is not valid anymore, and has to be replaced with a weighted least square (wls) procedure [1, 2]. The need for weighted least square procedures has been recognized already around 1800 by mathematicians like Laplace, Legende, and Gauss [3], but was, initially, not pursued because of complex numerics. With the advent of the computers in the 1950s/1960s numerical difficulties stopped to exist. Yet, weighted least squares was first included in the SPSS statistical software since 1998 (SPSS version 8) [4]. It is, currently, commonly applied in geometry, nature science, and social science [1, 2], but clinical applications have been few. Searching Medline we found one pulmonary physiology paper [5], one PET imaging paper [6], and one disease seasonality paper [7], but no treatment efficacy studies.

The current paper was written to familiarize the clinical research community with this relevant methodology. A simulated study of the effects of medicine dosages on the peak expiratory flows of 78 bronchial asthma patients was used. Step by step analyses in SPSS [4] together with the data file are given.

3 Example

A 78 patient simulated sample of the effect of different dosages of prednisone and beta agonist on peak expiratory flow in bronchial asthma was used. The investigators expected that, with increasing dosages of prednisone, the effect on peak expiratory flow was more variable. SPSS statistical software was applied. The data file is in Table 10.1. For convenience an SPSS data file, entitled "chap10peakexpiratoryflow. sav", is available on the internet at extras.springer.com.

> Command: Menu....Analyze....Regression....Linear....select: Dependent: enter peakflow.... Independent(s): enter prednisone, betaagonist....click Plots....select ZRESID as y-variable....ZPRED as x-variable....click Continue....click Save....select Standardized in Residuals....click Continue....click OK.

In the outcome sheets the R value of 0.763 is observed (Table 10.2 upper table), and the linear effects of the treatment dosages on the peakflow is in Table 10.2 (lower table). The prednisone dosages, are a statistically significant predictor of the peak expiratory flow, but, surprisingly, the beta agonists dosages are not. The plot of the standardized predicted values against the standardized residuals suggest the presence of heteroscedasticity: the spread of the residuals (y-axis) increase with increase of the predictors. This is not in agreement with the assumption of the linear ordinary linear regression model. We will return to the data file, which now contains a novel variable: ZRE_1 (the standardized residuals). We will use WLS for valid estimations.

> Command: Menu....Graphs....Char Builder....select Scatter/Dot....choose Simple Scatter....select the standardized residuals variable as the y-variable....select prednisone as the x- variable....click OK.

Figure 10.1 shows the plot of standardized prednisone values against the standardized residuals. The pattern is similar to that of the prednisone dosages against the outcome residuals (Fig. 10.2), and confirms that prednisone dosages are the cause of the heteroscedasticity. We will, subsequently, perform a WLS analysis.

> Command: Menu....Analyze....Regression....Weight Estimation.... select: Dependent: enter peakflow.... Independent(s): enter prednisone, betaagonist....select prednisone also as Weight variable....Power range: enter 0 through 5 by 0.5....click Options....select Save best weights as new variable....click Continue....click OK.

In the outcome sheets it is observed that the software has calculated likelihoods for different powers, and the best likelihood value is chosen for further analysis. When returning to the data file again a novel variable is added, the WGT_1 variable (the weights for the WLS analysis).

The next step is to perform again a linear regression, but now with the weight variable included.

> Command: Menu....Analyze....Regression....Linear.... select: Dependent: enter peakflow.... Independent(s): enter prednisone, betaagonist....select the weights for the wls analysis (the GGT_1) variable as WLS Weight....click Save....select Unstandardized in Predicted Values....deselect Standardized in Residuals....click Continue....click OK.

Table 10.1 Data file of example: the effect of different dosages of prednisone and beta agonists on peak expiratory flow in 78 patients with bronchial asthma

Pat No.	Prednisone mg/24 h	Peak flow ml/min	Beta agonist mg/24 h
1	29	1,40	174
2	15	2,00	113
3	38	0,00	281
4	26	1,00	127
5	47	1,00	267
6	28	0,20	172
7	20	2,00	118
8	47	0,40	383
9	39	0,40	97
10	43	1,60	304
11	16	0,40	85
12	35	1,80	182
13	47	2,00	140
14	35	2,00	64
15	38	0,20	153
16	40	0,40	216
17	15	0,40	75
18	31	1,00	231
19	32	0,20	116
20	36	0,20	315
21	41	0,00	248
22	10	0,20	61
23	48	0,20	420
24	27	0,60	185
25	45	0,60	270
26	29	0,00	143
27	46	0,40	187
28	20	0,60	136
29	54	1,20	303
30	10	1,80	83
31	26	0,40	106
32	11	0,40	65
33	35	0,20	73
34	58	1,40	440
35	23	0,80	110
36	19	0,00	134
37	24	0,00	123
38	31	0,20	187
39	28	0,20	91
40	29	1,40	174
41	15	2,00	113
42	38	0,00	281
43	26	1,00	127
44	47	1,00	267

(continued)

Table 10.1 (continued)

Pat No.	Prednisone mg/24 h	Peak flow ml/min	Beta agonist mg/24 h
45	28	0,20	172
46	20	2,00	118
47	47	0,40	383
48	39	0,40	97
49	43	1,60	304
50	16	0,40	85
51	35	0,20	182
52	47	0,20	140
53	35	2,00	64
54	38	0,20	153
55	40	0,40	216
56	15	0,40	75
57	31	1,00	231
58	32	0,20	116
59	36	0,20	315
60	41	0,00	248
61	10	1,80	61
62	48	1,80	420
63	27	0,60	185
64	45	0,60	270
65	29	0,00	143
66	46	0,40	187
67	20	0,60	136
68	54	1,20	303
69	10	1,80	83
70	26	0,40	106
71	11	0,40	65
72	35	0,20	73
73	58	1,40	440
74	23	0,80	110
75	19	0,00	134
76	24	0,00	123
77	31	0,20	187
78	28	0,20	91

The outcome table shows an R value of 0.846 (Table 10.3, upper table). It has risen from 0.763, and provides thus more statistical power. Table 10.3, lower table shows the effects of the two medicine dosages on the peak expiratory flows. The t-values of the medicine predictors have increased from approximately 10 and 0.5 to 14 and 3.2. The p-values correspondingly fell from 0.000 and 0.552 to respectively 0.000 and 0.002. Larger prednisone dosages and larger beta agonist dosages significantly and independently increased peak expiratory flows. After adjustment for heteroscedasticity, the beta agonist became a significant independent determinant of peak flow.

Table 10.2 Multiple linear regression with the two medicines as predictors and the peak flow as outcome

Model summary[b]

Model	R	R square	Adjusted R square	Std. error of the estimate
1	,763[a]	,582	,571	65,304

[a] Predictors: (Constant), beta agonist mg/24h, prednisone mg/day

[b] Dependent variable: peak expiratory flow

Coefficients[a]

Model		Unstandardized coefficients B	Std. error	Standardized coefficients Beta	t	Sig.
1	(Constant)	−22,534	22,235		−1,013	,314
	Prednisone mg/day	6,174	,604	,763	10,217	,000
	beta agonist mg/24h	6,744	11,299	,045	,597	,552

[a] Dependent variable: peak expiratory flow

Prednisone but not the beta agonist significantly increases the peak flows

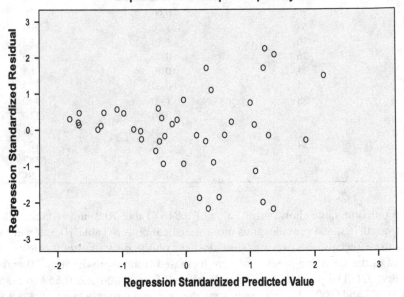

Dependent Variable: peak expiratory flow

Fig. 10.1 The plot of the standardized predicted values (1) against the standardized residuals (2) in this regression analysis suggests the presence of heteroscedasticity: the larger (1) the wider the spread in (2)

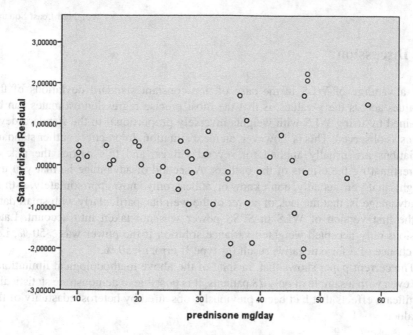

Fig. 10.2 The heteroscedasticity is mainly caused by the effect of the prednisone variable: wit larger prednisone dosages there is much more spread in the outcome data than with small dosages. The prednisone variable can, thus, be used for correcting the heteroscedasticity in this example

Table 10.3 The weighted linear regression is more powerful. The r square value has increased from 0.764 to 0.845

Model summary[b,c]

Model	R	R square	Adjusted R square	Std. error of the estimate
1	,846[a]	,716	,709	,125

[a] Predictors: (Constant), beta agonist mg/24h, prednisone mg/day

[b] Dependent variable: peak expiratory flow

[c] Weighted Least Squares Regression–Weighted by Weight for peakflow from WLS, MOD_6 PREDNISONE**–3,500

Coefficients[a,b]

Model		Unstandardized coefficients		Standardized coefficients		
		B	Std. error	Beta	t	Sig.
1	(Constant)	5,029	7,544		,667	,507
	Prednisone mg/day	5,064	,369	,880	13,740	,000
	beta agonist mg/24h	10,838	3,414	,203	3,174	,002

[a] Dependent variable: peak expiratory flow

[b] Weighted Least Squares Regression–Weighted by Weight for peakflow from WLS, MOD_6 PREDNISONE**–3,500

The t-values of the medicine predictors have increased from approximately 10 and 0.5 to 14 and 3.2. The p-values correspondingly fell from 0.000 and 0.552 to 0.000 and 0.002. Larger prednisone dosages and larger beta agonist dosages significantly and independently increase peak expiratory flows

4   Discussion

The advantage of WLS in the case of non-constant standard deviations of the y-values across the x-values, is that the most precise regression estimates can be obtained by using WLS with weights inversely proportional to the standard deviations as observed. This is, however, an ideal situation. In practice, outlier standard deviations are usually applied for several values, and this carries the risk of overestimating the effects of the outliers. A second disadvantage is, that you use weights that you, actually, don't know or, at best, only know approximately. A third disadvantage is, that the lack of power of the weights, particularly with small data. In the first version of WLS in SPSS power was not taken into account. Later versions only accepted weighted variance solution if the power was >50 %, i.e., the chance of a false negative result (or type II error) <50 %.

The current paper shows that, in spite of the above methodological limitations, and even with a sample of only 78 patients, it is possible to demonstrate statistically significant effects that had been, previously, obscured by heteroscedasticity of the y-value.

5   Conclusions

1. The current paper shows that, even with a sample of only 78 patients, WLS is able to demonstrate statistically significant linear effects that had been, previously, obscured by heteroscedasticity of the y-value.
2. The most precise regression estimates can be obtained by using weighted least squares linear regression with weights inversely proportional to the standard deviations as observed.
3. This is, however, an ideal situation. In practice, outlier standard deviations are usually applied for several values, and this carries the risk of overestimating the effects of the outliers.
4. Another disadvantage is that you use weights that you, actually, don't know or, at best, only know approximately.
5. A final disadvantage is the lack of power of the weights, particularly with small data. SPSS only accepts weighted variance solutions, if the power is >50 %, i.e., and the chance of a false negative result (or type II error) <50 %.

References

1. Anonymous (2013) Weighted least squares. www.itl.nist.gov/div898/handbook. 9 June 2013
2. Anonymous (2009) Extending linear regression: weighted least squares, heteroscedasticity, local polynomial regression. 36–350 Data Mining. 23 Oct 2009. Pittsburgh, PA, USA, www.stat.cmu. edu. 9 June 2013

3. Nievergelt Y (2000) A tutorial history of least squares. J Comput Appl Math 121:37–72
4. SPSS Statistical Software (2013) www.spss.com. 9 June 2013
5. Ferreira J, Vasconcelos F, Tierra-Criollo C (2011) A case study of applying weighted least squares to calibrate a digital maximum respiratory pressures measuring system. In: Applied biomedical engineering. John Hopkins University, Baltimore
6. Fessler J (1994) Penalized weighted least squares image reconstruction for PET. IEEE Trans Med Imaging 13:290–299
7. Brookhart MA, Rothman KJ (2008) Simple estimators of the intensity of seasonal occurrence of monocytic leucemia. BMC Med Res Methodol 8:67–71

Chapter 11
Multiple Response Sets

1 Summary

1.1 Introduction

The analysis of multiple questions about a single disease/condition is generally analyzed with frequency tables for each question separately.

1.2 Objective

Multiple response methodology is another possibility, and it is available in SPSS statistical software. It provides summary tables enabling to visualize trends in the data.

1.3 Methods

A hypothesized 812 patient health survey was used to compare this machine learning methodology with that of traditional frequency tables.

1.4 Results

Unlike traditional frequency table, multiple response tables demonstrated various trends that could be selected for formal trend tests.

T.J. Cleophas and A.H. Zwinderman, *Machine Learning in Medicine: Part Three*, DOI 10.1007/978-94-007-7869-6_11, © Springer Science+Business Media Dordrecht 2013

1.5   Conclusions

1. The answers to a set of multiple questions about a single underlying disease/
   condition can be assessed as multiple dimensions of a complex variable.
2. Multiple response methodology is adequate for the purpose.
3. The most important advantage of the multiple response methodology versus
   traditional frequency table analysis is, that it is possible to observe relevant
   trends, and similarities in the data.
4. A disadvantage is that only summaries but no statistical tests are given, but
   observed trends can, of course, be, additionally, tested statistically with formal
   trend tests.
5. Unlike machine learning methods like factor analysis, discriminate analysis and
   cluster analysis that are kind of black box methods and hard for investigators to
   check, multiple response methodology is mathematically very simple, and, yet,
   hard to perform without a computer.
6. This chapter shows that machine learning needs not necessarily be complicated.
7. Multiple response sets are adequate for visualizing trends in clinical data.

2   Introduction

It is convenient to assess the answers to a set of multiple related qualitative
questions about a single underlying disease/condition as multiple dimensions of a
complex variable. This method, called multiple response sets, enables to a simultaneous assessment of the answers, visualizing patterns of response and visualizing
effects of other variables, like personal characteristics, comorbidities,
comedications and other personal features on these pattern responses. Up to
20 questions can be simultaneously assessed. The method is particularly useful if
the numbers of answers is much less than the numbers of questions, and if there are
many patients who did not answer any of the questions (here called the missing
cases). These kinds of data are very common in survey research like patient health
surveys in health care. In econometry/sociometry the method is used for the
assessment of consumer questionnaires. Similar information can be obtained from
usual frequency tables, but the information given is less compact and less complete,
and it is given in the form of separate tables for each question and separate crosstabs
for the interaction of each question with other variables like personal characteristics. The most important advantage of the multiple response methodology is that, by
an overall simultaneous assessment of multiple questions, it is possible to observe
relevant trends and similarities in the data. A disadvantage is that only summaries
but no statistical tests are given, but observed trends can, of course, be additionally
tested statistically with, e.g., formal trend tests.

SPSS started in 1968, and multiple response analysis is available since 1990 [1],
but, although widely used in econometry/sociometry [2], is little used in clinical

research. The current paper was written as an introduction to the method for the medical community. A hypothesized example of health questionnaire data was used. A step by step analysis was given for the convenience of investigators planning to use this methodology themselves.

3 Example

A hypothesized 811 person health questionnaire addressed the reasons for visiting general practitioners (gps) in 1 month. The data is entitled "chap11healthmultipleresponseset.sav", and can be downloaded from the internet at extras.springer.com. Nine qualitative questions addressed various aspects of health as primary reasons for visits. SPSS statistical software was used to analyze the data.

> Command: Analyze....Multiple Response....Define Variable Sets....move "ill feeling, alcohol, tiredness, cold, family problem, mental problem, physical problem, social problem" from Set Definition to Variables in Set....Counted Values enter 1....Name enter "health"....Label enter "health"....Multiple Response Set: click Add....click Close.... click Analyze....Multiple Response....click Frequencies ....move $health from Multiple Response Sets to Table(s)....click OK.

The output consists of two tables. Table 11.1 shows the number of patients who answered yes to at least one question. Of all visitants 25.6 % did not answer any question, here called the missing cases. In Table 11.2 the letter N gives the numbers of yes-answers per question, "Percent of Cases" gives the yes-answers per question in those who answered at least once (missing data not taken into account), and "Percent" gives the percentages of these yes-answers per question. The gp consultation burden of mental and physical problems was about twice the size of that of alcohol and weight problems. Tiredness and social problems were in-between.

In order to assess these data against all visitants, the missing cases have to be analyzed first.

> Command: Transform....Compute Variable....Target Variable: type "none"....Numeric Expression: enter "1-max(illfeeling, ..., social problem)" ....click Type and Label... .LabelL enter "no answer"....click Continue....click OK....Analyze....Multiple Response ....Define Variable sets....click Define Multiple Response Sets....click $health....move "no answer" to Variables in Set....click Change....click Close.

The data file now contains the novel "no answer" variable and a novel multiple response variable including the missing cases but the latter is not shown. It is now also possible to produce crosstabs with the different questions as rows and other variables like personal characteristics as columns. In this way the interaction with the personal characteristics can be assessed.

> Command: Analyze....Multiple Response....Multiple Response Crosstabs....Rows: enter $health....Columns: enter ed (= level of education)....click Define Range....Minimum: enter 1....Maximum: enter 5....Continue....Click Options....Cell Percentages: click Columns.... click Continue....click OK.

Table 11.1 The number of
patients who answered yes to
at least one question. Of all
visitants 25.6 % did not
answer any question, here
called the missing cases

Case summary						
	Cases					
	Valid		Missing		Total	
	N	Percent	N	Percent	N	Percent
$health[a]	722	74,4 %	248	25,6 %	970	100,0 %

[a]Dichotomy group tabulated at value 1

Table 11.2 The letter N
gives the numbers of
yes-answers per question,
"Percent of Cases" gives the
yes-answers per question in
those who answered at least
once (missing data not taken
into account), and Percent
gives the percentages of these
yes-answers per question

$health frequencies				
		Responses		
		N	Percent	Percent of cases
health[a]	illfeeling	391	12,9 %	54,2 %
	alcohol	242	8,0 %	33,5 %
	weight problem	214	7,1 %	29,6 %
	tiredness	300	9,9 %	41,6 %
	cold	389	12,8 %	53,9 %
	family problem	395	13,0 %	54,7 %
	mental problem	401	13,2 %	55,5 %
	physical problem	409	13,5 %	56,6 %
	social problem	293	9,7 %	40,6 %
Total		3,034	100,0 %	420,2 %

[a]Dichotomy group tabulated at value 1

The output table (Table 11.3) gives the results. Various trends are observed. E.g., there is a decreasing trend of patients not answering any question with increased levels of education. Also there is an increasing trend of ill feeling, alcohol problems, weight problems, tiredness and social problems with increased levels of education. If we wish to test whether the increasing trend of tiredness with increased level of education is statistically significant, a formal trend test can be performed.

Command: Analyze....Descriptive Statistics....Crosstabs....Rows: enter tiredness.... Columns: enter level of education....click Statistics....mark Chi-square....click Continue....click OK.

In the output (Table 11.4) the chi-square tests are given. The linear-by-linear association data show a chi-square value of 184.979 and 1 degree of freedom. This means that a statistically very significant linear trend with $p < 0.0001$ is in these data.

Also the interaction of health problems with all of the other variables including gender, age, marriage, income, period of constant address or employment can be similarly analyzed.

Table 11.3 Crosstabs with the different questions as rows and other variables like personal characteristics as columns

$health*ed crosstabulation

		Level of education					
		No highschool	Highschool	College	University	Completed university	Total
health[a]	illfeeling	Count					
		45	101	87	115	43	391
		% within ed					
		27,6 %	43,3 %	50,9 %	60,2 %	81,1 %	
	alcohol	Count					
		18	55	52	83	34	242
		% within ed					
		11,0 %	23,6 %	30,4 %	43,5 %	64,2 %	
	weight problem	Count					
		13	51	43	82	25	214
		% within ed					
		8,0 %	21,9 %	25,1 %	42,9 %	47,2 %	
	tiredness	Count					
		10	55	71	122	42	300
		% within ed					
		6,1 %	23,6 %	41,5 %	63,9 %	79,2 %	
	cold	Count					
		71	116	85	96	21	389
		% within ed					
		43,6 %	49,8 %	49,7 %	50,3 %	39,6 %	
	family problem	Count					
		75	118	84	93	25	395
		% within ed					
		46,0 %	50,6 %	49,1 %	48,7 %	47,2 %	
	mental problem	Count					
		78	112	91	94	26	401
		% within ed					
		47,9 %	48,1 %	53,2 %	49,2 %	49,1 %	
	physical problem	Count					
		78	123	87	95	26	409
		% within ed					
		47,9 %	52,8 %	50,9 %	49,7 %	49,1 %	
	social problem	Count					
		11	67	68	11	36	293
		% within ed					
		6,7 %	28,8 %	39,8 %	58,1 %	67,9 %	
	no answer	Count					
		39	29	13	6	2	89
		% within ed					
		23,9 %	12,4 %	7,6 %	3,1 %	3,8 %	
Total		Count					
		163	233	171	191	53	811

Percentages and totals are based on respondents

[a]Dichotomy group tabulated at value 1

*Sign of multiplication (here health questions by educational levels)

ed = educational level

Table 11.4 Formal trend test testing whether an increasing trend of tiredness is associated with increased levels of education

Chi-square tests

	Value	df	Asymp. sig. (2-sided)
Pearson chi-square	185,824[a]	4	,000
Likelihood ratio	202,764	4	,000
Linear-by-linear association	184,979	1	,000
N of valid cases	811		

[a]0 cells (,0 %) have expected countless than 5. The minimum expected count is 19,61

4   Discussion

An advantage of the multiple response method unlike traditional multiple frequency tables is, that all of the variables are simultaneously given in a single analysis. For illustration traditional frequency tables of the health variables are given.

> Command: Descriptive Statistics....Frequencies....Variables: enter the variables between "illfeeling" to "no answer"....click Statistics....click Sum....click Continue....click OK.

The output is in the underneath ten tables (Table 11.5). It is pretty hard to observe trends across the tables. Also redundant information as given is not helpful for overall conclusion about the relationships between the different questions.

Machine learning methodologies like cluster analysis, factor analysis, and discriminant analysis have been demonstrated to offer data analyses with relevant results, but the problem is often that the methods are rather complicated and the computer is used as a kind of black box: you have to believe the results but do not understand every step the computer has taken. In contrast, multiple response methodology is also a machine learning tool, but in contrast to the above methods it does not require sophisticated algebra and is simple to understand. Nonetheless it is very helpful to trend analysis of large datasets and is hard to replace with any other methods. Obviously, machine learning methods need not necessarily be complicated. The multiple response method can only be used for explorative research and statistical testing requires additional methods like chi-square trend tests.

5   Conclusions

1. The answers to a set of multiple questions about a single underlying disease/condition can be assessed as multiple dimensions of a complex variable.
2. Multiple response methodology is adequate for the purpose.

Table 11.5 The output of the descriptive statistics: frequency tables of health variables

Illfeeling

		Frequency	Percent	Valid percent	Cumulative percent
Valid	No	420	43,3	51,8	51,8
	Yes	391	40,3	48,2	100,0
	Total	811	83,6	100,0	
Missing	System	159	16,4		
Total		970	100,0		

Alcohol

		Frequency	Percent	Valid percent	Cumulative percent
Valid	No	569	58,7	70,2	70,2
	Yes	242	24,9	29,8	100,0
	Total	811	83,6	100,0	
Missing	System	159	16,4		
Total		970	100,0		

Weight problem

		Frequency	Percent	Valid percent	Cumulative percent
Valid	No	597	61,5	73,6	73,6
	Yes	214	22,1	26,4	100,0
	Total	811	83,6	100,0	
Missing	System	159	16,4		
Total		970	100,0		

Tiredness

		Frequency	Percent	Valid percent	Cumulative percent
Valid	No	511	52,7	63,0	63,0
	Yes	300	30,9	37,0	100,0
	Total	811	83,6	100,0	
Missing	System	159	16,4		
Total		970	100,0		

Cold

		Frequency	Percent	Valid percent	Cumulative percent
Valid	No	422	43,5	52,0	52,0
	Yes	389	40,1	48,0	100,0
	Total	811	83,6	100,0	
Missing	System	159	16,4		
Total		970	100,0		

Family problem

		Frequency	Percent	Valid percent	Cumulative percent
Valid	No	416	42,9	51,3	51,3
	Yes	395	40,7	48,7	100,0
	Total	811	83,6	100,0	
Missing	System	159	16,4		
Total		970	100,0		

(continued)

Table 11.5 (continued)

Mental problem

		Frequency	Percent	Valid percent	Cumulative percent
Valid	No	410	42,3	50,6	50,6
	Yes	401	41,3	49,4	100,0
	Total	811	83,6	100,0	
Missing	System	159	16,4		
Total		970	100,0		

Physical problem

		Frequency	Percent	Valid percent	Cumulative percent
Valid	No	402	41,4	49,6	49,6
	Yes	409	42,2	50,4	100,0
	Total	811	83,4	100,0	
Missing	System	159	16,4		
Total		970	100,0		

Social problem

		Frequency	Percent	Valid percent	Cumulative percent
Valid	No	518	53,4	63,9	63,9
	Yes	293	30,2	36,1	100,0
	Total	811	83,6	100,0	
Missing	System	159	16,4		
Total		970	100,0		

No answer

		Frequency	Percent	Valid percent	Cumulative percent
Valid	,00	722	74,4	89,0	89,0
	1,00	89	9,2	11,0	100,0
	Total	811	83,6	100,0	
Missing	System	159	16,4		
Total		970	100,0		

3. The most important advantage of the multiple response methodology versus traditional frequency table analysis is that it is possible to observe relevant trends and similarities in the data.
4. A disadvantage is that only summaries but no statistical tests are given, but observed trends can, of course, be, additionally, tested statistically with formal trend tests.
5. Unlike machine learning methods like factor analysis, discriminate analysis and cluster analysis, that are kind of black box methods and hard for investigators to check, multiple response methodology is mathematically very simple, and, yet, hard to perform without a computer.
6. The methodology shows that machine learning needs not necessarily be complicated.

References

1. Anonymous (2013) Corporate history-SPSS. www.spss.com. 6 Jan 2013
2. Hox J (2002) Multilevel analysis, techniques and applications. LEA Publishers, Mahwah

Chapter 12
Complex Samples

1 Summary

1.1 Background

The research of entire populations is costly and obtaining information from selected representative samples instead is more time- and cost-efficient. However, this method is generally biased due to selection bias. Complex sample technology is better suitable for that purpose, because it produces largely unbiased population estimates. It is little used in clinical research.

1.2 Objective

To familiarize the clinical research community with this novel methodology.

1.3 Methods

The hypothesized health scores of a 9,678 member population were assessed using both traditional simple random sampling and complex sampling methodologies. SPSS statistical software was applied.

1.4 Results

Both methodologies produced virtually the same summary statistics including means, correlation coefficients and ratios. However, the confidence intervals and standard

T.J. Cleophas and A.H. Zwinderman, *Machine Learning in Medicine: Part Three*,
DOI 10.1007/978-94-007-7869-6_12, © Springer Science+Business Media Dordrecht 2013

errors of the novel methodology were generally 3–4 times larger. Nonetheless, the analyses remained adequately powerful to demonstrate statistically significant differences.

1.5   Conclusions

Compared to traditional simple random sampling and entire population assessment the novel complex sampling methodology offers a number of advantages.

1. Complex samples is a cost-efficient method for analyzing target populations that are large and topographically heterogeneous.
2. It is time-efficient.
3. It offers greater scope and deeper insight, because specialized equipments are feasible.
4. It offers greater accuracy, because higher quality personnel and better training are feasible.
5. Traditional analysis of limited samples from heterogeneous target populations is a biased methodology, because each individual selected is given the same probability. In complex sampling this bias is adjusted by assigning appropriate weights to each individual included.
6. Current statistical software offers the possibility to conduct various types of regression analyses of complex samples including linear, logistic and Cox proportional hazard modeling.
7. Complex sampling is adequate for obtaining unbiased samples from demographic data.

2   Introduction

Population scores like financial, physical, mental, social and many other types of scores are the subject of study not only by governments and public authorities, but also by commercial institutions like pharmaceutical companies, health organizations and other research groups [1, 2]. Objectives include prediction purposes, the allocation of resources and others. The research of entire populations is laborious and obtaining information from representative samples instead is more time- and cost-efficient [1–3]. However, this method is generally biased, because each individual selected is given the same probability of being selected. Complex sample technology is particularly suitable for that purpose, because it produces largely unbiased population estimates [1–3]. This, however, requires special sampling techniques taking into account the different probabilities of individuals being included in a population-based survey. It is a computationally intensive method that calculates weighting factors for the individuals included. It was invented by William Cochran, professor of statistics at Harvard University, MA, US, in 1953 [4], but it took half a century, before it was to be implemented in major statistical software programs. It is now available in statistical programs like SPSS statistical software, since version 12, launched July 2004 [5], making it accessible to clinical investigators, particularly, those involved in surveys, like postmarketing drug surveillance data. However, to date no such studies have been published. Using the search term "complex samples" and "clinical studies" Google Scholar provides, in addition to nationwide public surveys, a multitude of analytical chemistry/biochemistry papers, but, otherwise, no clinical papers. This is, however, probably a matter of time.

The current paper was written to familiarize the clinical research community with this novel methodology. It uses a hypothesized example of a 9,678 member population health scores, and is supposed to assess the improvements in the past few years. The results of complex sample analyses and those of traditional analyses are compared. SPSS statistical software is applied for all of the analyses. For the benefit of students step be step analyses will be given.

3 A Real Data Example

An interesting real data example is given by SPSS [5] in its tutorial program. In the year 2000 the National Institute of Health in the USA wished to study health parameters of the USA citizens including smoking habits, vitamin and mineral supplies, multivitamin consumption, body weight, daily exercise information, and herbal supplies. The study could include about 0.3 billion of inhabitants, and census information was used to obtain most of the values of different states, city districts, and even townships and neighborhoods. However, little was known about the health parameters. It was decided to randomly sample 30,000 inhabitants throughout the country as a representative sample of the entire population, and these data would have to be used for comparisons between states, cities and other subgroups. However, it was duly recognized that different parts of the country would have different probabilities of being included in the sample. First, the states were not equally sized, and, thus, larger states had a larger chance of including individuals. Second, the sampled individuals were taken from different cities and city districts, and these were again different in probability of being included. For these differences probability corrections had to be performed and a correction factor, otherwise called weighting factor, had to be added to each individual in the sample prior to data analysis. This complex analysis is hard to accomplish without complex sampling procedures, and step by step analyses are given in SPSS [5].

4   Some Theory

Health scores, including measures of physical, mental and social health are increasingly considered important to estimate public health [6]. If in one county 40 % has a low health score and in another equally large county 60 %, then on average 50 % has a low health score. If the first county is larger than the second, e.g. 1.5 times larger (with similar population density), then we have 1.5 times larger chance that an individual from the 40 % low scores is sampled. This would mean that, instead of an average of 50 % low health scores for the two counties,

$$(1/2 \times 40 + 1/2 \times 60)/2 = 50 \ \%,$$

the following average will be measured:

$$(3/5 \times 40 + 2/5 \times 60)/2 = 48 \ \%.$$

This result is 2 % smaller, and this is due to the difference in size of the two counties. Complex sample methodology adjusts these kinds of effects by adding appropriate weights to the individual data. However, with experimental data, uncertainty should be taken into account, and this is also true for the weights to be added as a multiplication factor to the individuals' data. This complicates statistical analyses. Different mathematical methods are available for adjusting the biased estimations [1]. The replication method randomly selects a set of sub-samples from the sampled data and overall estimates are computed from them. The Jackknife method works similarly and calculates means and variances by repeatedly deleting one measured value. Both are Monte Carlo methods and can be applied without the need to take account of theoretical data distribution patterns. They are, respectively, used by default in SPSS with proportional and numeric data. Taylor series makes use of the algebraic phenomenon that any function f(x) can be expressed as the sum of another function f(a) and its derivative times $(x - a)$ [2]. It enables to account and compute the variances of ratio data and weighted ratios. We should add that computations are further complicated by the repeated nature of many observations in population studies, requiring paired analyses, and accounting, not only the variances but also the covariances in the data.

5   Example

Prior health scores of a 9,678 member population recorded some 5–10 years ago were supposed to be available as well as topographical information. We wish to obtain information of the current versus the prior health scores, using complex samples methodology. For that purpose the information of the entire data plus additional information on the current health scores from as random sample of 1,000 from this population were used. The region consisted of four counties, 88 townships and 613 neighborhoods. First, a sampling plan was designed.

Then, a random sample of 1,000 was taken and additional information was obtained and included in the data file. The latter data file plus the sampling plan were, then, used for various complex samples analyses. Also the results of traditional and the complex samples analyses were compared. The SPSS modules complex samples (cs) descriptives, cs general linear model, and cs ratios were applied as well as the appropriate modules for the traditional analyses.

6 Sampling Plan (Table 12.1)

A sampling plan of the above population data is designed using SPSS. Open in extras.springer.com the database entitled "chap12healthscores_cs.sav". Then command:

> click Analyze....Complex Samples.... Select a sample.... click Design a sample, click Browse: select a map and enter a name, e.g., healthscore_cs.plan....click Next....Stratify by: select county....Clusters: select township....click Next...Type: Simple Random Sampling....click Without replacement....click Next....Units: enter Counts....click Value: enter 4....click Next....click Next....click (Yes, add stage 2 now)....click Next...Stratify by: enter neighbourhood....next...Type: Simple random sampling.... click Without replacement....click Next....Units: enter proportions....click Value: enter 0,25....click Next....click Next....click (No, do not add another stage now)....click Next...Do you want to draw a sample: click Yes....Click Custom value....enter 123.... click Next....click External file, click Browse: select a map and enter a name, e.g., healthscores_cssample ....click Save....click Next....click Finish.

In the output table a summary of the sampling plan is given (Table 12.1). In the original data file the weights of 1,006 randomly sampled individuals are given. These had to be used for further analyses, and additional information on current health scores of these individuals had to be obtained and included in the cs sample file. In the maps selected above we find two new files, (1) entitled "chap12healthscore_cs.plan" containing the weighting procedures (this map can not be opened, but it can in closed form be entered whenever needed during further complex samples analyses of these data), and (2) entitled "chap12healthscores_ssample.sav" containing 1,006 randomly selected individuals from the main data file. The latter data file is first completed with current health scores before the definitive analysis. Only of 974 individuals the current information could be obtained, and these data were added as a new variable (see "chap12healthscores_cssample.sav" at extras.springer.com). Also (1) has for convenience been made available at extras.springer.com.

Table 12.1 Population data summary

Population	9,678 cases
Counties	4
Townships	88
Neighborhoods	613
Stage 1 sampling plan	
	The counties are the strata,
	The townships are the clusters
	4 clusters/stratum
Stage 2 sampling plan	
	The neighborhoods are the strata
	The cases are the clusters (clusters of one)
	A proportion of 0.2 of the cases clustered/stratum

7   Complex Samples Analyses

We now use the above data files (1) and (2) for further analyses. The averages of the current and prior health scores (I), their linear relationship level (II), and their ratios (III) will be assessed and tested.

(I) Averages of the current and prior health scores.

Open the data file (2). Then command:

Analyze....Complex Samples....Descriptives....click Browse: select the appropriate map and enter healthscore_cs.plan....click Continue...Measures: enter last healthscore, enter curhealthscore....Subpopulations: enter County....click Statistics: mark Mean, 95 % Confidence interval, Design effect....click OK.

Table 12.2 (upper part) gives the means and 95 % confidence intervals. Also design effects are given (not shown). The design effects are sometimes relevant because they are the ratios of the variances of the complex sampling method versus those of the traditional, otherwise called simple random sampling (srs), method. In the given example the ratios are mostly 3–4, which means that the uncertainty of the complex samples methodology is 3–4 times larger than that of the traditional method. However, this reduction in precision is compensated for by the removal of biases due to the use of inappropriate probabilities used in the srs method.

The Table 12.2 (lower part) gives the srs data obtained through the usual commands (Analyze, Descriptive Statistics, Explore, Dependent list (last and curhealthscores), Factor list (County), Statistics (mark Descriptives)). It is remarkable to observe that, although the two methods produce virtually the same means, the confidence intervals are very different. E.g., for the Northern region, curhealthscores), the 95 % confidence intervals went from 11.7–19.6 to 14.9–16.4, which means that the complex samples results estimates were about three times wider.

Table 12.2 Means of health scores per county; complex sample analysis (upper table) and traditional simple random sampling (srs) analysis (lower table)

County			Estimate	95 % confidence interval	
				Lower	Upper
Eastern	Mean	last healthscore	19,3040	18,9277	19,6803
		curhealthscore	24,5659	21,0591	28,0726
"Southern	Mean	last healthscore	17,6714	16,9828	18,3601
		curhealthscore	24,5764	20,8233	28,3295
"Western	Mean	last healthscore	11,8569	11,2562	12,4576
		curhealthscore	14,9585	14,4260	15,4910
Northern	Mean	last healthscore	10,1317	9,6571	10,6063
		curhealthscore	15,6330	11,7072	19,5588

			Estimate	95 % confidence interval
Eastern	mean	last	19,3013	19,0373–19,5653
		cur	24,5651	23,7960–25,3452
Southern		last	17,669	17,2885–18,0512
		cur	24,6023	23,7761–25,4285
Western		last	11,7100	11,3559–12,0642
		cur	14,9553	14,4485–15,4620
Northern		last	10,1281	9,8899–10,3662
		cur	15,65451	14,8993–16,3908

The complex sample means are similar to the traditional means. However, the standard errors are substantially larger, sometimes 3–4 times. The current scores tend to be larger than the old scores

(II) Linear relationship level between the current and prior health scores.

Open the data file (2). Then command:

Analyze….Complex Samples….General Linear Model….click Browse: select the appropriate map and enter healthscore_cs.plan….click Continue…Dependent variable: enter curhealthscore….Covariates: enter last healthscores….click Statistics: mark Estimates, 95 % Confidence interval, t-test….click OK.

It may take a few seconds. Table 12.3 (upper part) gives the correlation coefficient and the 95 % confidence intervals. The Table 12.3 (lower part) gives the srs data obtained through the usual commands (Analyze, Regression, Linear, Dependent (curhealthscore), Independent (s) (last healthscore), OK). It is remarkable to observe the differences between the two analyses. The correlation coefficients are largely the same but their standard errors are respectively 0.158 and 0.044. The t-value of the complex sampling analysis equals 5.315, while that of the traditional analysis equals no less than 19.635. Nonetheless, the reduced precision of the

Table 12.3 Linear regression of health scores, complex sample analysis (upper table) and traditional simple random sampling (srs) analysis (lower table)

Parameter estimates[a]

Parameter	Estimate	Std. error	95 % confidence interval		Hypothesis test		
			Lower	Upper	t	df	Sig.
(Intercept)	8,151	2,262	3,222	13,079	3,603	12,000	,004
lasthealthscore	,838	,158	,494	1,182	5,315	12,000	,000

[a] Model: curhealthscore = (Intercept) + lasthealthscore

Coefficients[a]

Model		Unstandardized coefficients		Standardized coefficients	t	Sig.
		B	Std.error	Beta		
1	(Constant)	7,353	,677		10,856	,000
	last healthscore	,864	,044	,533	19,635	,000

[a] Dependent variable: curhealthscore

The complex samples general linear model is given with last appraisal as independent and current appraisal as dependent variable. The old scores is a very significant predictor of the new scores

complex sampling analysis did not produce a statistically insignificant result, and, in addition, it was, of course, again adjusted for inappropriate probability estimates.

(III) Ratios of the current and prior health scores.

Open the data file (2). Then command:

Analyze. ...Complex Samples. ...Ratios. ...click Browse: select the appropriate map and enter healthscore_cs.plan. ...click Continue. ..Numerators: enter last curhealthscore. ...Denominator: enter last healthscore. ...Subpopulations: entere County. ...click Statistics: mark Standard error, Confidence interval (enter 95 %), Design effect. ...click Continue. ...click OK.

Table 12.4 (upper part) gives the overall ratio and the ratios per county plus 95 % confidence intervals. Also design effects are given. The design effects are the ratios of the variances of the complex sampling method versus that of the traditional, otherwise called simple random sampling (srs), method. In the given example the ratios are mostly 3–4, which means that the uncertainty of the complex samples methodology is 3–4 times larger than that of the traditional method. However, this reduction in precision is compensated for by the removal of biases due to the use of inappropriate probabilities used in the srs method.

The Table 12.4 (lower part) gives the srs data obtained through the usual commands (Analyze, Descriptive Statistics, Ratio, Numerator (curhealthscore), Denominator (lasthealthscore), Group Variable (County), Statistics (means, confidence intervals etc.). Again the ratios of the complex samples and traditional analyses are rather similar, but the confidence intervals are very different. E.g., the 95 % confidence intervals of the Northern County went from 1.172 to 1.914 in

Table 12.4 Ratios of health scores per county: complex sample analysis (upper table) and traditional simple random sampling (srs) analysis (lower table)

Ratios 1

Numerator	Denominator	Ratio estimate	Standard error	95% confidence interval		Design effect
				Lower	Upper	
curhealthscore	last healthscore	1,371	,059	1,244	1,499	17,566

Ratios 1

County	Numerator	Denominator	Ratio estimate	Standard error	95% confidence interval		Design effect
					Lower	Upper	
Eastern	curhealthscore	last healthscore	1,273	,076	1,107	1,438	12,338
"Southern	curhealthscore	last healthscore	1,391	,100	1,174	1,608	21,895
"Western	curhealthscore	last healthscore	1,278	,039	1,194	1,362	1,518
Northern	curhealthscore	last healthscore	1,543	,170	1,172	1,914	15,806

Ratio statistics for curhealthscore / last healthscore

Group	Mean	95% confidence interval for mean		Price related differential	Coefficient of dispersion	Coefficient of variation
		Lower bound	Upper bound			Median centered
Eastern	1,282	1,241	1,323	1,007	,184	24,3%
"Southern	1,436	1,380	1,492	1,031	,266	33,4%
"Western	1,342	1,279	1,406	1,051	,271	37,7%
Northern	1,613	1,525	1,702	1,044	,374	55,7%
Overall	1,429	1,395	1,463	1,047	,285	41,8%

Ratios of scores of individuals in different parts of a region of current versus previous scores. Although the mean values were virtually similar to those from the traditional analysis, the SEs (standard errors of the complex sample assessments were 4–5 times the size of those from the traditional computations. The ratios given underscore the Table 12.1 data

the complex samples, and from 1.525 to 1.702 in the traditional analysis, and was thus over three times wider in the former analysis.

In addition to the statistics given above, other complex samples statistics are possible, and they can be equally well executed in SPSS, that is if the data are appropriate. If you have a binary outcome variable (dichotomous) available, then logistic regression modeling is possible, if an ordinal outcome variable (polytomous) is available, ordinal regression, if time to event information is on the data, complex samples Cox regression can be performed.

8   Discussion

Over 50 years ago William Cochran, professor of statistics Harvard University, Cambridge MA US, pointed out that our knowledge is largely based on samples [4]. However, there are bad and good samples. E.g., the report of someone travelling a country for 10 days is bad compared to the report of someone studying the country for 15 years. Nonetheless, even the latter report is based on fragments of knowledge of the country. Traditionally, the best information of a target population seems to be provided by the assessment of the entire population. However, this is costly and laborious, and broad data often suffer from flaws like low quality samples and missing data. Cochran was an advocate of limited samples, and summarized the following advantages.

1. Reduced costs.
2. Greater speed.
3. Greater scope and deeper insight, because of highly specialized equipments.
4. Greater accuracy, also because of higher quality personnel and better training.

It is currently recognized that the technique of complex sampling introduced by him has brought additional advantages. One is that traditional analysis of limited samples from heterogeneous target populations is a biased methodology, because each individual selected is given the same probability, and the spread in the data is, therefore, severely underestimated. In complex sampling this bias is adjusted for by assigning appropriate weights to each individual included.

Another advantage is the possibility to conduct various types of regression analyses including linear, logistic and Cox proportional hazard modeling of adjusted complex sample data, and to compare the results with those of traditional analyses, and quantitatively assess the differences.

Complex sampling has some disadvantages. First, it is, of course, less efficient than a traditional srs analysis of a complex sample, because it yields estimates of lower precision.

Second, with traditional sampling prior sample size calculations enable to predict the statistical power of a study. With complex samples this is not impossible. However, it is pretty hard, because the power is not only depends on the magnitude of the outcome, but also on the individual weights of the outcome variables and the interactions between weights and the outcome. The best power is obtained if the variables in the population strata and the complex samples are proportional with one another, but also this may be hard to realize with random sampling. However, survey research is mostly explorative, and starting the analysis with a complex sample consisting of just a small proportion of the target population, e.g., 0.10 and adding another 0.05 if results were not yet statistically significant, is, methodologically, no problem.

The current paper shows that the spread in the data with the complex sampling method was 3–4 times wider than it was with the simple random sampling method. Nonetheless, p-values were very small, like 0.0001, and one could argue that the data analyses given were somewhat overpowered, and that a (much) smaller complex sample from the target population in our example would also have been adequate for the null-hypotheses.

9 Conclusions

We conclude the following. Compared to traditional simple random sampling and entire population assessment the novel complex sampling methodology offers a number of advantages.

1. Complex samples is a cost-efficient method for analyzing target populations that are large and heterogeneously topographically distributions.
2. It is time-efficient.
3. It offers greater scope and deeper insight, because specialized equipments are feasible.
4. It offers greater accuracy, because higher quality personnel and better training are feasible.
5. Traditional analysis of limited samples from heterogeneous target populations is a biased methodology, because each individual selected is given the same probability, and the spread in the data is, therefore, generally underestimated. In complex sampling this bias is adjusted for by assigning appropriate weights to each individual included.
6. Current statistical software offers the possibility to conduct various types of regression analyses of complex samples including linear, logistic and Cox proportional hazard modeling.

References

1. Anonymous (1988) Statistical methods for analyzing a complex sample survey. Public Health Service, Centers of Disease Control, National Center for Health Statistics, Ed by National Institute of Health, Washington, DC
2. Lee ES, Forthofer RN (2006) Analyzing complex survey data, 2nd edn. www.sagepub.com. 24 Apr 2013
3. Rafferty A (2013) Introduction to complex sample design in UK Government Surveys. ESDS (Economic and Social Data Service) Government web site. www.esds.ac.uk/government. 24 Apr 2013
4. Cochran WG (1953) Sampling techniques. John Wiley & Sons, New York
5. SPSS Statistical Software (2013) www.spss.com. 20 Apr 2013
6. Ware JE (1987) Standards for health measures. J Chron Dis 40:473–478

Chapter 13
Runs Test

1 Summary

1.1 Background

R-square values are often used to test the appropriateness of diagnostic models.

However, in practice, a pretty large r-square value (squared correlation coefficients) may be observed even if data do not systematically follow the model selected.

1.2 Objective

To assess whether the runs test is a better alternative to the traditional r-square test for addressing the differences between the data and the model in non-linear regression modeling.

1.3 Methods

A real data example was given comparing quantity of care with quality of care scores.

1.4 Results

Unlike the r-square statistic, the runs test was able to differentiate between more and less appropriate curvilinear regression models with p-values <0.02 versus = 0.40 respectively.

T.J. Cleophas and A.H. Zwinderman, *Machine Learning in Medicine: Part Three*, DOI 10.1007/978-94-007-7869-6_13, © Springer Science+Business Media Dordrecht 2013

1.5   Conclusions

1. The runs test is appropriate both for (1) goodness of fit testing of frequency distributions, and (2) testing whether fitted theoretical curves are systematically different or not from a given data set.
2. The function (1) may sometimes be assessed with more power by traditional goodness of fit tests, like the Kolmogorov-Smirnov test.
3. The function (2) is in regression models traditionally assessed with r-square tests. However, the runs test is more appropriate for the purpose, as demonstrated in the example of this chapter. This is, because the runs test assesses the entire data pattern, rather than mean distances between data and model.
4. The runs test can be performed with a pocket calculator, but it is available in most major software programs including SPSS statistical software.

2   Introduction

In 1968 James Vandiver Bradley, a statistician at Aerospace Medical Research Laboratories, Lackland Air Force Base, Texas, published a book entitled Distribution-free statistical concepts [1]. In Chap. 12 of this book the authors covered a novel test for determining whether data differ systematically from a theoretical model. The test has now been widely used by econometrists [2], sociometrists [2] and psychologists [3], but like many machine learning tools little by clinicians, who traditionally very much rely on prospective blinded placebo controlled clinical trials. This is a pity, since many clinical observations, particularly, longitudinal observations are hard to analyze with traditional parallel group statistics, and can be more easily assessed with non-linear models, like curvilinear regression models, and auto-correlation methods [4, 5]. The runs test can be used with any data pattern and has advantages. It does not model data itself, but rather tests whether already selected models are or are not in agreement with the patterns as observed in the data. And, so, it does not select the models, but rather tests the appropriateness of the model selected by other methods like, e.g., regression methods. A run is a series of consecutive points with a residual of the same sign (positive or negative). If a best fit model for your data is calculated with, e.g., regression analysis, a perfect fit is rarely obtained. The distances of the data from the best fit regression model can be split into subsequent runs of positive and negative deviations. For different sizes of data sets, different numbers of runs have been demonstrated to be compatible with randomness. If too many or too few runs are observed, the null hypothesis of randomness is rejected, and it is concluded that the data differ systematically from the model as calculated. Runs tests are different from r-square tests. The latter measures the strength of association of the data with the model, while the runs tests measures the entire pattern of the data file as compared with that of the model: the data may be pretty distant from the model, but, as soon as runs occur regularly, the pattern of the model may still be appropriate to describe the data. Also, in practice, a pretty large r-square value may be observed even if data do not systematically follow the model. We, therefore, believe that the runs statistic is a better device to test the appropriateness of a diagnostic model than the r-square statistic.

The current paper was written to familiarize clinical investigators with the test. We will use a real data example. Step by step analyses will be given.

3 Example

Doctors were assessed for the relationship between their quantity and quality of care. The quantity of care was estimated with the numbers of daily interventions like endoscopies and small operations per doctor, the quality of care with quality of care scores. The data file is given in Table 13.1, and is also available as "chap13runstest.sav" on the internet at extras.springer.com. The relationship seemed not to be linear, and curvilinear regression in SPSS was used to find the

Table 13.1 The quantity of care estimated as the numbers of daily interventions like endoscopies and small operations per doctor tested against the quality of care scores	Quantity of care	Quality of care
	19,00	2,00
	20,00	3,00
	23,00	4,00
	24,00	5,00
	26,00	6,00
	27,00	7,00
	28,00	8,00
	29,00	9,00
	29,00	10,00
	29,00	11,00
	28,00	12,00
	27,00	13,00
	27,00	14,00
	26,00	15,00
	25,00	16,00
	24,00	17,00
	23,00	18,00
	22,00	19,00
	22,00	20,00
	21,00	21,00
	21,00	22,00

Quantity of care = numbers of daily interventions per doctor, Quality of care = quality of care scores

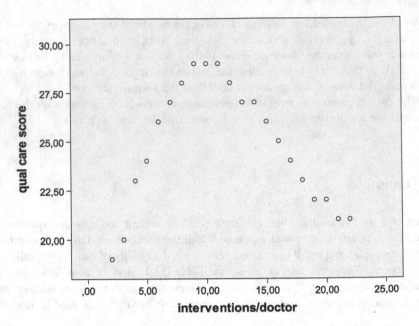

Fig. 13.1 Scattergram of the data from Table 13.1

best fit curve to describe the data and eventually use them as prediction model. First, we will make a graph of the data.

Command: Analyze....Graphs....Chart builder....click: Scatter/Dot....Click quality of care and drag to the Y-Axis....Click Intervention per doctor and drag to the X-Axis....OK.

Figure 13.1 shows the scattergram of the data. A non-linear relationship is indeed suggested. The curvilinear regression option in SPSS may be helpful to find the best fit model.

Command: Analyze....Regression....Curve Estimation....mark: Quadratic, Cubic.... mark: Display ANOVA Table....OK.

Figure 13.2 shows the quadratic (best fit second order, parabolic, relationship) and cubic (best fit third order, hyperbolic, relationship) as produced by the software program.

The Table 13.2 shows the test statistics of quadratic and cubic modeling of the data file from Table 13.1: The least squares were excellent both for the quadratic and the cubic model with p-values <0.0001. From these results it is hard to choose which of the two provides the best fit model for making predictions from these data. The runs test is used to find out whether the two models differ systematically from the data.

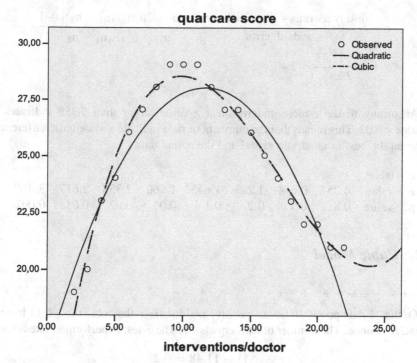

Fig. 13.2 The quadratic (best fit second order, parabolic, relationship) and cubic (best fit third order, hyperbolic, relationship) model from the data from Table 13.1 is produced by the software program

Table 13.2 Test statistics of quadratic and cubic modeling of the data file from Table 13.1: The least squares were excellent both for the quadratic and the cubic model with p-values <0.0001

Model summary and parameter estimates

Dependent variable:qual care score

Equation	Model summary					Parameter estimates			
	R square	F	df1	df2	Sig.	Constant	b1	b2	b3
Quadratic	,866	58,321	2	18	,000	16,259	2,017	−,087	
Cubic	,977	236,005	3	17	,000	10,679	4,195	−,301	,006

From these results it is hard to choose the best fit model for making predictions from these data The independent variable is interventions/doctor

3.1 Quadratic Model

− − + − + + + + + + + − − − − − − − − − − +++

Of the 21 data points 11 have a positive residue from the quadratic model, 10 a negative residue. The number of runs equals 6.

The z-statistic is used to statistically test this number of runs (n_1 = the numbers of positive residues, n_2 = the number of negative residues):

$$z = \frac{observed\ runs - expected\ runs}{standard\ error} = \frac{6 - [2n_1n_2/(n_1 + n_2)] + 1}{\sqrt{(n_1 + n_2)^2\ (n_1 + n_2 - 1)}}$$

$$z = \frac{6 - 11.48}{2.28} = 2.40$$

According to the z-table underneath a z-value larger than 2.358 indicates a p-value <0.02. This means that the numbers of runs indicate a systematic difference between the best fit quadratic model and the actual data.

z − table								
z − value	0.254	0.674	1.283	1.645	1.960	2.358	2.617	3,160
p − value	0.8	0.5	0.2	0.1	0.05	0.02	0.01	0.002

3.2 Cubic Model

$$+ - + - - - - + + + + - + + - - - - - + - +$$

Of the 21 data points 10 have a positive residue from the cubic model, 11 have a negative residue. The number of runs equals 11. The z-test is performed like above.

$$z = \frac{11 - 11.48 = 0.2}{2.28}$$

According to the above z-table the p-value is larger than 0.8. This means that this number of runs indicates that no systematic difference from the best fit cubic model is observed in these data. The best fit cubic model is a better prediction model for these data than the best fit quadratic model is.

4 Runs Test in SPSS [6]

For those with little affinity to pocket calculator activities a runs test is available in SPSS statistical software. For that purpose the data file has to be slightly changed. The positive and negative residues from the selected best fit models have to be added as separate variables (Table 13.3).

Command: Analyze....Nonparametric tests....Runs Test....move the runsquadratic model residues variable to Test Variable List....click Options....click Descriptives....click Continue....click Cut Point....mark Median....click OK.

The Table 13.4 gives the output table of the runs test for the best fit quadratic model. A statistically significant runs test indicates that the quadratic model is systematically different from the data. When the similar procedure is followed for

Table 13.3 Like in Table 13.1 the quantity of care estimated as the numbers of daily interventions like endoscopies and small operations per doctor tested against the quality of care scores (first and second columns)

Quantity of care	Quality of care	Residues quadratic model	Residues cubic model
19,00	2,00	0,00	1,00
20,00	3,00	0,00	0,00
23,00	4,00	1,00	1,00
24,00	5,00	0,00	0,00
26,00	6,00	1,00	0,00
27,00	7,00	1,00	0,00
28,00	8,00	1,00	0,00
29,00	9,00	1,00	1,00
29,00	10,00	1,00	1,00
29,00	11,00	1,00	1,00
28,00	12,00	1,00	1,00
27,00	13,00	0,00	0,00
27,00	14,00	0,00	1,00
26,00	15,00	0,00	1,00
25,00	16,00	0,00	0,00
24,00	17,00	0,00	0,00
23,00	18,00	0,00	0,00
22,00	19,00	0,00	0,00
22,00	20,00	1,00	1,00
21,00	21,00	1,00	0,00
21,00	22,00	1,00	1,00

The third and fourth column present the residues from respectively the best fit quadratic and the cubic models of the data (instead of the signs − and + the values 0 and 1 have to be used in SPSS)

Table 13.4 The output table of the runs test for the best fit quadratic model

Runs test

	Runs quadratic model
Test value[a]	1,00
Cases < test value	10
Cases >= test value	11
Total cases	21
Number of runs	6
Z	−2,234
Asymp. sig. (2-tailed)	,026
Exact sig. (2-tailed)	,022
Point probability	,009

[a]Median

the best fit cubic model, again a runs test output table is produced (Table 13.5). As the median was 0 a runs test could not be performed. Instead it was performed with the mean of the data. The z-value was small and statistically insignificant. The data were thus systematically not-different from the best fit cubic model. The cubic model was a better predicting model for the data than the quadratic model.

Table 13.5 The output table of the runs test for the best fit cubic model

Runs test 2	
	Runs cubic model
Test value[a]	,4762
Cases < test value	11
Cases >= test value	10
Total cases	21
Number of runs	11
Z	,000
Asymp. sig. (2-tailed)	1,000
Exact sig. (2-tailed)	1,000
Point probability	,165

[a]Mean

5   Discussion

The runs test is currently often called the Wald-Wolfowitz test after Abraham Wald, mathematician, Vienna, Austria, 1950, and Jacob Wolfowitz, statistician, New York University, New York, NY, USA, 1970, who recommended the test as a general method for checking any random hypothesis [7]. As such it can be used not only to test whether a function fits well to a data set, but also to test the randomness of frequency distributions. In this way it is similar to the traditional goodness of fit tests, like the chi-square goodness of fit and the Kolmogorov Smirnov goodness of fit tests, although the latter may be sometimes statistically somewhat more powerful [8].

The current study shows, that the runs test can also be used as a method for assessing whether a data set is systematically different from a best fit selected mathematical model. If so, the selected model should not be applied for making sound predictions. With regression models the r square test is often used to test whether the data are significantly closer to the selected model than could happen by chance, but large and statistically very significant r-squares may be observed even if data are pretty distant from the selected model. In the example given, according to the r-square tests both the quadratic and cubic models were appropriate prediction models. However, according to the runs tests, only the cubic model was appropriate for such purpose. We, therefore, believe that runs tests are a better alternative to the traditional r-square tests for finding appropriate predictions models from curvilinear regression models.

6   Conclusions

1. the runs test is appropriate both for (1) goodness of fit testing of frequency distributions, and (2) testing whether fitted theoretical curves are systematically different or not from a given data set.

2. The function (1) may sometimes be assessed with more power by traditional goodness of fit tests, like the Kolmogorov-Smirnov test.
3. The function (2) is in regression models traditionally assessed with r-square tests. However, the runs test is more appropriate for the purpose, because large r-square value do not exclude poor systematic data fit, and because the runs test assesses the entire pattern in the data, rather than mean distances between data and model.
4. The runs test can be performed with a pocket calculator, but it is available in most major software programs including SPSS statistical software.

References

1. Bradley JV (1968) Chapter 12, The runs test. In: Distribution-free statistical concepts. Prentice Hall Inc., Englewood Cliffs
2. Anonymous (2013) Runs test for detecting non-randomness. www.itl.nist.gov.div898/hand book/eda/section3/eda35d.htm. 3 June 2013
3. Maddux CD (2012) SPSS for windows-the runs test for randomness. http://wolfweb.unr.edu/ homepage/maddux/stat/cep741/runwin.html. 3 June 2012
4. Cleophas TJ, Zwinderman AH (2013) Chapter 14, Multivariate analysis of time-series. In: Cleophas TJ, Zwinderman AH (eds) Machine learning part two. Springer, Heidelberg
5. Cleophas TJ, Zwinderman AH (2012) Chapter 15, Curvilinear estimation. In: Cleophas TJ, Zwinderman AH (eds) SPSS for starters part 2. Springer, Heidelberg
6. SPSS Statistical Software (2013) www.spss.com. 3 June 2013
7. Anonymous (2013) Wald-Wolfowitz test. http://en.wikipedia.org.wiki/Wald%E2%80%93Wolf owitz_runs_test. 4 June 2013
8. Cleophas TJ, Zwinderman AH (2011) Chapter 42, Testing clinical trials for randomness. In: Cleophas TJ, Zwinderman AH (eds) Statistics applied to clinical research, 5th edn. Springer, Heidelberg, pp 469–478

Chapter 14
Decision Trees

1 Summary

1.1 Background

Decision trees are widely used in econo-/sociometry for decision analysis of real world problems. It is little used in clinical research.

1.2 Objective

To assess its performance in predicting health outcomes.

1.3 Methods

Simulated data examples with both a binary and a continuous outcome variable were used. SPSS statistical software was applied.

1.4 Results

In the examples given the results were statistical more powerful than were similar analyses in multiple linear and logistic regression with Wald statistics of 207 versus 100, and t-statistics of 16.6 versus 12.2.

T.J. Cleophas and A.H. Zwinderman, *Machine Learning in Medicine: Part Three*, DOI 10.1007/978-94-007-7869-6_14, © Springer Science+Business Media Dordrecht 2013

1.5   Conclusions

1. Decision trees assess the effects of predictor variables on numbers of events and other health outcomes, and is comparable with multiple logistic/linear regression.
2. The advantages over regression modeling include its flexibility and lack of the various limitations of regression modeling like the assumption of non-collinearity, no confounding, and no interaction between predictors, and the requirement of homoscedasticity, Gaussian pattern around the dependent variable, and linear relationship.
3. It is, therefore wrongly, little used in clinical research.
4. In the examples given it provided more sensitivity and precision both with binary and with continuous outcome variables than the regression models appropriate for the data did.
5. Decision trees is adequate for predicting both continuous and discrete health outcomes.

2   Introduction

Decision trees assess the effects of predictor variables on numbers of events and other health outcomes. It is very comparable with multiple logistic/linear regression. Multiple logistic regression similarly assesses the risk of an event in sub-groups, but uses odds ratios instead of total numbers. Multiple linear regression similarly predicts the reduction or improvement of an outcome level in individuals with certain predictors, but uses the best fit linear equations, instead of the means of subgroups.

Although widely applied, there is an analytical problem with multiple logistic/linear regression. It, principally, assumes that predictors are entirely independent of one another. E.g., the risk of a myocardial infarct is determined by multiple factors, like gender, weight, age, cholesterol, lifestyle, etc. However, why should all of these factors be independent of one another [1]. A nice thing about decision trees is, that interaction between predictors is not an issue. The tree consists of multiple partitions with the strongest association between independent and dependent variable at each subsequent partition.

Decision trees has a pretty long history. The classification and regression tree (CRT) method for continuous outcome variables is a method comparable with ROC (receiver operated characteristic) methodology, but the result is adjusted for the magnitudes of the samples. It is invented by Claude Shannon, computer scientist at Bell Laboratories Massachusetts, USA, in the early 1950s [2]. The chi-square automatic interaction detection (CHAID) method is a method suitable for decision trees with a binary outcome variable. It was invented by Ross Quinlan, computer scientist at Sydney University, Australia [3].

Perlich et al. [4] summarized the advantages of decision trees versus the traditional multiple regression. In addition to the lack of problems with interaction between exposure variables, computational difficulties with large data are rarely observed.

Like other machine learning methods as factor analysis and cluster analysis, although widely used for econo-/sociometry and computer science, it is little used in clinical research. When searching Medline we found four gynecology papers [5–8], two cardiology papers [9, 10], two psychiatry papers [11, 12], one nuclear medicine [13], one adverse drug effect paper [14], one infectious disease paper [15], one world health issue paper [16], and one surgery paper [17], but, otherwise, few papers addressing specific health outcome issues [18].

The current chapter using simulated examples assesses the efficacy of decision analysis for predicting both continuous and discrete health outcomes, like treatment efficacy levels and event frequencies. SPSS statistical software is used for data analysis [19].

3 Some Terminology

3.1 Decision Tree

Tree-based classification model with single dependent variable and multiple predictors.

3.2 Decision Tree Validation

Each computation produces a single best fit tree: tree validation is accomplished with (1) cross validation (the study sample is split into multiple subsamples that are estimated for misclassification risks), (2) split-sample validation (a hold out sample obtained from the entire dataset is used to assess the quality of the modeled tree) [20].

3.3 Entropy Method (Lit: Entropy = Measure of Rate of Transfer)

The entropy method makes use of equations formerly applied to estimate the amount of energy loss in thermodynamics. Like ROC (receiver operated characteristic) curves it optimizes node splitting, but a pleasant thing is that it is adjusted for magnitude of the samples [21].

3.4   Gains Number and Percentage (in CHAID)

Number of subgroup cases in each terminal node with a positive outcome. The percentage is the ratio of gains numbers and all patients with a positive outcome in the entire file ($\times 100$ %).

3.5   Index

Ratio of response in node and response in entire data ($\times 100$ %). This value is an measure of how far the observed percentage of responders differs from the expected percentage of responders if the predictors had no effect.

3.6   Node

(1) the parent node is the entire sample of patients (cases) in your data file (root node), (2) the internal nodes are subgroups partitioned (otherwise called segmented, categorized, stratified) according to some independent variables, (3) the terminal nodes are the final nodes in a tree, they are the nodes at which the tree stops growing [20–24].

3.7   Node Impurity (in CRT)

Measure of misclassification in internal nodes estimated with maximal log likelihood of outcome if predictor variable follows Gaussian pattern.

3.8   Pruning

Removing relatively small nodes to simplify the tree, it is only possible with CRT trees.

3.9   Response (in CHAID)

The ratio of the gains number and total number of cases in a node ($\times 100$ %).

3.10 Tree Growing Methods

The tree growing methods are (1) for binary outcomes chi-squared automatic interaction detection (CHAID)[3], here the parent nodes can be split into two or more child nodes, (2) for continuous outcomes classification and regression trees (CRT) [22], here parent nodes are split only into two child nodes.

4 Decision Trees with a Binary Outcome (CHAID Analysis), Example

In a 1004 patient data file of risk factors for myocardial infarct a chi-squared automatic interaction (CHAID) model is used for analysis. The data file is entitled "chap14infarct_rating.sav', and is on the internet at extras.springer.com. The file is opened and we command.

> Command: Classify....Tree....Dependent Variable: enter infarct rating....Independent Variables: enter age, cholesterol level, smoking, education, weight level....Growing Method: select CHAID....click Categories: Target mark yes....Continue....click Output: mark Tree in table format....Criteria: Parent Node type 200, Child Node type 100.... Continue....click again Output: Statistics mark Gain, mark Index....Continue....click Save: mark Terminal node number, Predicted value, Predicted probabilities....click Continue....OK.

The Fig. 14.1 gives the decision tree of the chi-squared automatic interaction detection method. The Cholesterol level is the best predictor of the infarct rating. For low cholesterol the cholesterol level is the only significant predictor of infarction: only 35.5 % will have an infarction. In the medium and high cholesterol groups age is the next best predictor. In the elderly with medium cholesterol smoking contributes considerably to the risk of infarction. In contrast, in the younger with high cholesterol those with normal weight are slightly more at risk of infarction than those with high weights. Table 14.1 give the statistics of the tree model.

For each node (subgroup) the number of cases, the chi-square value, and level of significance is given. A p-value <0.05 indicates that the difference between the 2×2 or 3×2 tables of the paired nodes are significantly different from one another. All of the p-values were very significant.

Table 14.2 gives the gives the gains obtained by the model. Only terminal nodes are listed. In the two gain columns the numbers and percentages of patients with an infarct are given. In the index column ratios of percentages of patients with an infarction and the percentage of an infarction in the entire population is listed. E.g., 126.0 % = 100/79.4, and 123.3 % = 97.9/79.4. Two graphs further explain the tables, the cumulative gains and index charts (Fig. 14.2). The cumulative gains

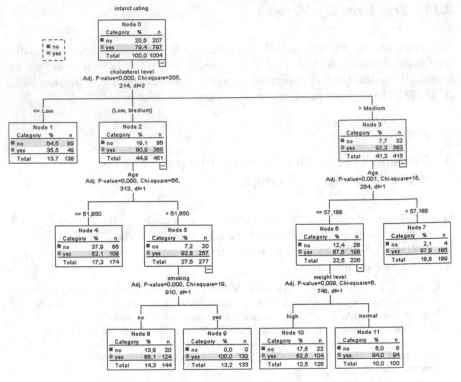

Fig. 14.1 Chi-squared automatic interaction detection (CHAID) decision tree model used for the analysis of the data from first example

chart always starts at 0 and ends at 100 %. The steeper the curve, the better the model. The cumulative index chart tends to start above 100 % and descends until 100 % is reached.

The risk and classification tables in Table 14.3 indicate that the category infarction predicted by the model is wrong in 0.166 = 16.6 % of the cases. A correct prediction of 83.4 % is fine. However, in those without an infarction no infarction is predicted in only 43.0 % of the cases.

When returning to the original data file we will observe 4 new variables, (1) the terminal node number, (2) the predicted outcome yes/no infarction for each case, (3, 4) the predicted probabilities that a case is in the infarction subgroup (or not). The latter variables are very significant predictors of infarction in the binary logistic regression with a Wald statistic of 207.886 (Table 14.4, upper table). This statistic is better than each of the statistics of multiple logistic regression with infarction as outcome and the risk factors as predictors (best Wald value for cholesterol level 100.561), (Table 14.4 lower table). This would mean that the decision tree model provides a better fit for the data than simple multiple logistic regression does.

Table 14.1 The tree table

Tree table

Mode	No		Yes		Total		Predicted category	Parent node	Primary independent variable				
	N	Percent	N	Percent	N	Percent			Variable	Sig.[a]	Chi-square	df	Split values
0	207	20,6 %	797	79,4 %	1004	100,0 %	yes						
1	89	64,5 %	49	35,5 %	138	13,7 %	no	0	cholesterol level	,000	205,214	2	<= Low
2	86	19,1 %	365	80,9 %	451	44,9 %	yes	0	cholesterol level	,000	205,214	2	(Low, Medium]
3	32	7,7 %	383	92,3 %	415	41,3 %	yes	0	cholesterol level	,000	205,214	2	>Medium
4	66	37,9 %	108	62,1 %	174	17,3 %	yes	2	Age	,000	65,313	1	<=51,580
5	20	7,2 %	257	92,8 %	277	27,6 %	yes	2	Age	,000	65,313	1	>51,850
6	28	12,4 %	198	87,6 %	226	22,5 %	yes	3	Age	,001	15,264	1	<=57,188
7	4	2,1 %	185	97,9 %	189	18,8 %	yes	3	Age	,001	15,264	1	>57,188
8	20	13,9 %	124	86,1 %	144	14,3 %	yes	5	smoking	,000	19,910	1	no
9	0	,0 %	133	100,0 %	133	13,2 %	yes	5	smoking	,000	19,910	1	yes
10	22	17,5 %	104	82,5 %	126	12,5 %	yes	6	weight level	,009	6,746	1	high
11	6	6,0 %	94	94,0 %	100	10,0 %	yes	6	Weight level	,009	6,746	1	normal

For each node (subgroup) the number of cases, the chi-square value, and level of significance is given. A p-value <0.05 indicates that the difference between the 2 × 2 or 3 × 2 tables of the paired nodes are significantly different from one another. All of the p-values were very significant

Growing method: CHAID

Dependent variable: infarct rating

[a]Bonferroni adjusted

Table 14.2 The gains
obtained by the model

Gains for nodes						
	Node		Gain			
Node	N	Percent	N	Percent	Response	Index
9	133	13,2 %	133	16,7 %	100.0 %	126,0 %
7	189	18,8 %	185	23,2 %	97,9 %	123,3 %
11	100	10,0 %	94	11,8 %	94,0 %	118,4 %
8	144	14,3 %	124	15,6 %	86,1 %	108,5 %
10	126	12,5 %	104	13,0 %	82,5 %	104,0 %
4	174	17,3 %	108	13,6 %	62,1 %	78,2 %
1	138	13,7 %	49	6,1 %	35,5 %	44,7 %

Only terminal nodes are listed. In the two gain columns the numbers and percentages of patients with an infarct are given. In the
index column ratios of percentages of patients with an infarction
and the percentage of an infarction in the entire population is listed.
E.g., 126.0 % = 100/79.4, and 123.3 % = 97.9/79.4
Growing method: CHAID
Dependent variable: Infarct rating

5   Decision Trees with a Continuous Outcome (CRT Analysis), Example

For decision trees with continuous outcome the classification and regression tree
(CRT) model is applied. An example is given. A 953 patient simulated data file is
used of various predictors of ldl (low-density-lipoprotein)-cholesterol reduction
including weight reduction, gender, sport, treatment level, diet. The file is in extras.
springer.com and is entitled "chap14tree_ldl_reduction.sav". The file is opened.

> Command: Analyze….Classify…Tree.…Dependent Variable: enter ldl_reduction.…
> Independent Variables: enter weight reduction, gender, sport, treatment level, diet.…
> Growing Methods: select CRT.…click Criteria: enter Parent Node 300, Child Node
> 100.…click Output: Tree mark Tree in table format.…Rules mark Generate classification
> rules.…mark Export rules to a file.…File: enter G:\chap14ldl_scores.sps.…Browse to
> navigate to a location in your computer.…click Continue.…click OK.

The output sheets show the classification tree (Fig. 14.3). Only weight reduction
and sport significantly contributed to the model, with the overall mean and standard
deviation dependent variable ldl cholesterol in the parent (root) node. Weight
reduction with a cut-off level of 1.3 units is the best predictor of ldl reduction.
In the little weight reduction group sport is the best predictor. In the low sport level
subgroup again weight reduction is a predictor, but here there is a large difference
between weight gain (<-1.5 units) and weight loss (>-1.5 units).

In order to assess whether the model provides an adequate fit for the data, the
within node variance is used as estimate for the variability in the data caused by
error. It equals 0.552 (Table 14.5). The total variance is found by calculating the
standard deviation of the root node (parent node), $2.162^2 = 4.674$. The proportion
of the total variance caused by error equals $0.552/4.674 = 0.118$. The proportion of

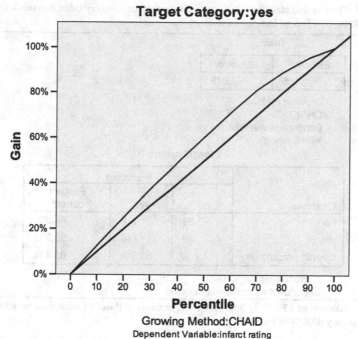

Growing Method:CHAID
Dependent Variable:infarct rating

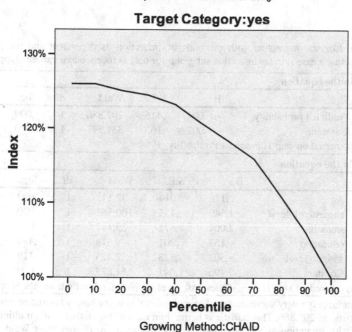

Growing Method:CHAID
Dependent Variable:infarct rating

Fig. 14.2 The cumulative gains and index charts. The cumulative gains chart always starts at 0 and ends at 100 %. The steeper the curve, the better the model. The cumulative index chart tends to start above 100 % and descends until 100 % is reached

Table 14.3 The risk and classification tables indicate that the category infarction predicted by the model is wrong in 0.166 = 16.6 % of the cases

Risk

Estimate	Std. error
,166	,012

Growing method:
CHAID
Dependent variable:
infarct rating

Classification

	Predicted		
Observed	no	yes	Percent correct
no	89	118	43,0%
yes	49	748	93,9%
Overall percentage	13,7%	86,3%	83,4%

Growing method: CHAID
Dependent variable: infarct rating

A correct prediction of 83.4 % is fine. However, in those without an infarction no infarction is predicted in only 43.0 % of the cases

Table 14.4 Logistic regression with the odds of infarction as dependent and the predicted probabilities that a case is in the infarction subgroup (or not) as independent variable (upper table)

Variables in the equation

		B	S.E.	Wald	df	Sig.	Exp(B)
Step 1[a]	Predicted probability_1	−6,004	,416	207,886	1	,000	,002
	Constant	3,007	,165	331,577	1	,000	20,217

[a]Variable(s) entered on step 1: PredictedProbability_1

Variables in the equation

		B	S.E.	Wald	df	Sig.	Exp(B)
Step 1[a]	Age	,118	,014	72,141	1	,000	1,125
	cholesterol_level	1,549	,155	100,561	1	,000	4,709
	smoking	2,004	,371	29,147	1	,000	7,420
	education	−,157	,201	,613	1	,434	,854
	weight_level	−,503	,323	2,425	1	,119	,605
	Constant	−7,496	1,041	51,877	1	,000	,001

[a]Variable(s) entered on step 1: Age, cholesterol_level, smoking, education, weight_level

The latter variable is a very significant predictor of infarction in the binary logistic regression with a Wald statistic of 207.886. This statistic is better than each of the statistics of a multiple logistic regression with infarction as outcome and the risk factors as predictors (best Wald value for cholesterol level 100.561) (lower table)

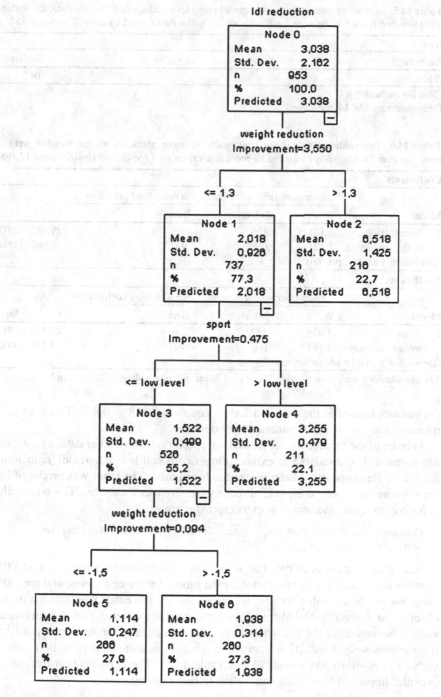

Fig. 14.3 The Classification and Regression Tree (CRT) of the 953 patient data file of predictors of ldl cholesterol reduction

Table 14.5 In order to assess whether the model provides an adequate fit for the data, the within node variance is used as estimate for the variability in the data caused by error. It equals 0.552

Risk

Estimate	Std. error
,552	,042

Growing method: CRT
Dependent variable: ldl reduction

Table 14.6 The predicted values are statistically stronger predicted by the variable weight reduction than the originally measured ldl reduction values with t-values of 16.606 versus 12.198

Coefficients[a]

Model	Unstandardized coefficients		Standardized coefficients		
	B	Std. error	Beta	t	Sig.
1 (Constant)	3,101	,106		29,382	,000
weight_reduction	1,131	,068	,947	16,606	,000

[a]Dependent Variable: pre_001

Coefficients[a]

Model	Unstandardized coefficients		Standardized coefficients		
	B	Std. error	Beta	t	Sig.
1 (Constant)	3,056	,152		20,120	,000
weight_reduction	1,195	,098	,907	12,198	,000

[a]Dependent Variable: ldl_reduction

The classification tree, thus, provided improved linear outcome values in this example

the variance caused by the tree model, thus, equals $1-0.118 = 0.882$. This is 88.2 % meaning that we have a considerably good model.

In order to use the tree model for making predictions from other data, a new data file is given. It is available at extras.springer.com entitled "chap14ldl_reduction. sav'. This file is opened. Also a syntax file is required. The latter was produced by the software and saved at the "G:" directory (see commands above). The syntax file is for convenience also stored at extras.springer.com.

Command: File....New....Syntax....type: INSERT FILE='chap14ldl_scores.sps' ....
Run....All.

Returning to the opened data file, we will now find two new variables: nod_001 contains the terminal nodes predicted by the model for the new cases, and pre_001 gives the predicted value for the ldl reduction for the case. It is interesting to observe the (considerable) differences between the predicted and the measures values. Nonetheless, the predicted values are statistically stronger predicted by the variable weight reduction than the originally measured ldl reduction values with t-values of 16.606 versus 12.198 Table 14.6). The classification tree, thus, provided improved linear outcome values in this example.

6 Discussion

Decision trees can be used for decision analysis of real world medical problems. In this chapter examples are given of both a model with a binary and with a continuous outcome variable. Decision tree analysis, particularly CRT trees, are also used for decision trees based on the best fit cut-offs between correct and incorrect classification for the purpose of predicting continuous health outcomes.

CRT is also used for validating diagnostic tests like ROC methods. However, it is more sensitive, because it is an entropy method taking the sample size of the cut-offs subgroups into account [21]. It is available in Breiman's CART statistical software program [22].

We have to admit, decision trees do have their limitations. They more easily suffer from overfitting than regression models, and, with small data, they are sometimes less robust [20–24].

The advantages are the flexibility and lack of the various limitations of regression: the assumptions of non-collinearity, no confounding, and no interaction between predictors, and the requirements of homoscedasticity, Gaussian pattern around the dependent variable, a linear relation between the y and x-variables [23].

The examples also show that in the examples given the results were statistical more powerful than similar analyses in multiple linear and logistic regression with test statistics of 207 versus 100 in the Wald tests for the binary outcome example, and of 16.6 versus 12.2 in the t-tests for the continuous outcome example.

Currently, the method of decision trees for continuous outcome variables is complemented with random forests, introduced by Breiman in 1999 [24]. They involve an ensemble of decision trees rather than a single one. An additional variable and bootstrap training samples are used. It turns out that the prediction rules from the forest procedures are more precise than those of a single tree, although the separate trees grown from a random forest may be worse predictors than the original best fit decision tree.

7 Conclusions

1. Decision trees assess the effects of predictor variables on numbers of events and other health outcomes. It is very comparable with multiple logistic/linear regression.
2. The advantages over regression modeling include its flexibility and lack of the various limitations of regression modeling like the assumption of non-collinearity, no confounding, and no interaction between predictors, and the requirement of homoscedasticity, Gaussian pattern around the dependent variable, a linear relationships.
3. It is, therefore wrongly, little used in clinical research.
4. In the examples given it provided more sensitivity and precision both with binary and with continuous outcome variables.

References

1. Cleophas TJ, Zwinderman AH (2012) Linear regression. In: Cleophas TJ, Zwinderman AH (eds) Statistics applied to clinical studies, 5th edn. Springer, Heidelberg, pp 199–203
2. Shannon CE (1951) Prediction and entropy of printed English. Bell Syst Tech J 30:50–64
3. Quinlan R (1999) Data mining from an A1 perspective. Data engineering 1999. In: Proceedings of the 15th international conference of data engineering, Sydney, Australia, p 186
4. Perlich C, Provost F, Simonoff JS (2003) Tree induction versus logistic regression. J Mach Learn 4:211–255
5. Babic S, Kokol P, Stiglic M (2000) Fuzzy decision trees in the support of breastfeeding. In: Proceedings 13th IEEE symposium on computer-based medical systems CBMS, Houston, pp 7–11
6. Zhang H, Legro R, Zhang J, Zhang L, Chen X, Huang H, Casson P, Schlaff W, Diamond M, Krawetz S, Coutifaris C, Brzyski R, Christman G, Santoro N, Eisenberg E, for the Reproductive Network (2010) Decision trees for identifying predictors of treatment effectiveness in clinical trials and its applications to ovulation in a study of women with polycystic ovary syndrome. Hum Reprod 25:2612–2621
7. Sims C, Meyn L, Caruana R, Rao R, Mitchell T, Krohn M (2000) Predicting caesarean delivery with decision tree models. Am J Obstet Gynecol 183:1198–1206
8. Tsien C, Kohane L, McIntosh N (2000) Multiple signal integration by decision tree induction to detect artifacts in the neonatal intensive care unit. Artif Intell Med 19:189–202
9. Sanders G, Hagerty C, Sonnenberg F, Hlatkey M, Owens D (2000) Distributed decision support using a web-based interface: prevention of sudden cardiac death. Med Decis Mak 19:157–166
10. Tsien C, Fraser H, Long W, Kennedy R (1998) Using classification tree and logistic methods to diagnose myocardial infarction. In: Proceedings 9th World Congress on Medical Informatics. MEDINFO'98, vol 52, Amsterdam, pp 493–497
11. Bonner G (2001) Decision making for health care professionals: use of decision trees within the community mental health setting. J Adv Nurs 35:349–356
12. Dantchev N (1996) Therapeutic decision trees in psychiatry. Encephale Revue de Psychiatrie Clinique Biologique et Therapeutique 22:205–214
13. Gambhir S (1999) Decision analysis in nuclear medicine. J Nucl Med 10:1570–1581
14. Jones J (2001) The role of data mining technology in the identification of signals of possible adverse drug reactions. Curr Ther Res 62:664–672
15. Ohno-Machado L, Lacson R, Massad E (2000) Decision trees and fuzzy logic: a comparison of models for the selection of measles vaccination strategies in Brazil. J Am Med Inform Assoc 9:625–629
16. Kokol P, Zorman M, Stiglic M, Malcic L (1998) The limitations of decision trees and automatic learning in real world medical decision making. In: Proceedings 9th World Congress on Medical Informatics. MEDINFO'98, vol 52, Amsterdam, pp 529–533
17. Letourneau S, Jensen L (1998) Impact of a decision tree on chronic wound care. Wound Ostomy Continence Nurs 25:240–247
18. Odgorelec V, Kokol P, Stiglic B, Rozman I (2002) Decision trees, an overview and their use in medicine. J Med Syst 26:445–463
19. SPSS Statistical Software (2013) www.spss.com. 15 July 2013
20. Anonymous (2011) Creating decision trees. BM Corporation, Armonk
21. Cleophas TJ, Zwinderman AH (2012) Binary partitioning. In: Cleophas TJ, Zwinderman AH (eds) Machine learning in medicine. Springer, Heidelberg, pp 79–86
22. Breiman L, Frieman JH, Olsen RA, Stone CJ (1984) Classification and regression trees. Chapman & Hall (Wadsworth Inc.), New York
23. Cleophas TJ, Zwinderman AH (2012) The limitations of linear regression. In: Cleophas TJ, Zwinderman AH (eds) Statistics applied to clinical studies, 5th edn. Springer, Heidelberg, p 176
24. Breiman L (2001) Random forests. Department of Statistics, University of California, Berkeley

Chapter 15
Spectral Plots

1 Summary

1.1 Background

In clinical research times series often show many peaks and irregular spaces.

Spectral plots is based on traditional Fourier analyses, and is available in the Forecasting module of SPSS statistical software. It can be helpful in this situation, and may be more sensitive than traditional autocorrelation analysis.

1.2 Objectives

To assess whether spectral analysis is sensitive for analysis even with wild data patterns.

1.3 Methods

A simulated data file of the monthly C reactive Protein (CRP), erythrocyte sedimentation rate (ESR), and percentage sick leave in a target population was used as an example. SPSS statistical software was used for analysis.

T.J. Cleophas and A.H. Zwinderman, *Machine Learning in Medicine: Part Three*,
DOI 10.1007/978-94-007-7869-6_15, © Springer Science+Business Media Dordrecht 2013

1.4   Results

In all of the examples annual periodicities were demonstrated by the spectral plot methodology, while the visual assessment of the data scatter-grams and the traditional autocorrelation analyses were inconclusive.

1.5   Conclusions

1. Times series often show many peaks and irregular spaces, and periodicity may not be evident. Traditional autocorrelation analysis has a limited sensitivity to detect periodicity.
2. Spectral analysis available in the Forecasting module of SPSS, and based on Fourier analyses was helpful in this situation, and was more sensitive than autocorrelation analysis.
3. In the examples given, unequivocal periodicities were demonstrated.
4. Smoothed curves obtained from spectral density analysis demonstrated that additional period effects did not exist.
5. The periodogram's variance does not decrease with increased sample sizes. However, smoothing using the spectral density function, is sample size dependent, and therefore, reduces this variance problem.

2   Introduction

In clinical research times series often show many peaks and irregular spaces, and the presence of periodicity may not be evident. Autocorrelation analysis is helpful to identify seasonal patterns, and was discussed in the first part of the current 3-volume book, entitled Machine Learning in Medicine [1]. However, autocorrelation has its limitations. Although the autocorrelation graphs may suggest the presence of seasonality, not only autocorrelation coefficients significantly larger than 0, but also smaller than 0 must be observed in order to conclude the unequivocal presence of a statistically significant seasonality. Spectral plots are helpful for support. It was invented by Schuster [2] in 1898, a physicist at the universities of Manchester UK and Heidelberg Germany, and is used to describe the dominating wavelet frequencies in a time series. Any time series can be described by a combination of cosine and sine waves of different periods and amplitudes. Fast form Fourier (FFT) transforms are used to find the best fit combination for a dataset, and are given by the function

$$f(x) = p + q_1 \cos(x) + \cdots + q_n \cos n(x) + r_1 \sin(x) + \cdots + r_n \sin n(x)$$

with $p, q_1 \ldots q_n$, and $r_1 \ldots r_n$ = constants for the best fit of the given data.

A periodogram has amplitude on the y-axis, but does not have time on the x-axis, but rather wavelet frequencies. Box and Jenkins [3] developed smoothing techniques to facilitate its use in time series analyses, and it is in its current version available in SPSS statistical software since 2007 (SPSS 16.0) [4].

The current chapter shows that spectral analysis is a welcome help if scatter-gram patterns and traditional autocorrelation are inconclusive, and you have clinical arguments for the presence of periodicity. Simulated data files of the monthly C reactive Protein (CRP), erythrocyte sedimentation rate (ESR), and percentage sick leave in a target population were used as examples. Step-by-step analyse are given in SPSS, not only with the help of the menu program, but also of the syntax program. We do hope that this chapter is helpful to clinical investigators puzzled by time series with many peaks and irregularities, particularly if they have sound clinical arguments for the presence of periodicity in the data.

3 Example

Simulated examples of 6 year monthly C reactive protein (CRP) levels (mg/l), erythrocyte sedimentation rate (ESR) (mm), and percentages sick leaves in a target population were used. The data (Fig. 15.1) display many peaks and irregularities in space, and the presence of periodicity is not unequivocal in the scatter-grams. Although the autocorrelation graphs (Fig. 15.2) suggest the presence of seasonality, in all of them this conclusion is based on a single value, i.e., the 12th month value. However, autocorrelation coefficients smaller than 0 are observed in none of the graphs. Not only autocorrelation coefficients significantly larger than 0 but also smaller than 0 must be observed in order to conclude the unequivocal presence of a statistically significant seasonality. Spectral plots are helpful for support. SPSS statistical software is used [3]. A data file is made available on the internet, entitled "chap15spectalanalysis.sav", at extras.springer.com.

> Command: Analyze.....Forecasting.....Spectral Analysis.....select CRP and enter into Variable(s).....select Spectral density in Plot.....click Paste.....change in syntax text: TSET PRINT-DEFAULT into TSET PRINT-DETAILED..... click Run.....click All.

In the output sheets the periodogram is observed (Fig. 15.3 upper part) with mean CRP values on the y-axis and frequencies on the x-axis. Of the peaks CRP-values observed the first one has a frequency of slightly less than 0.1. We assumed that CRP had an annual periodicity. Twelve months are in a year, months is the unit applied. As period is the inverted value of frequency a period of 12 months would equal a frequency of $1/12 = 0.0833$. An annual periodicity would produce a peak CRP-value with a frequency of $1/12 = 0.0833$. Indeed, the table in Fig. 15.3 (middle part) shows that at a frequency of 0.0833 the highest CRP value is observed. However, many more peaks are observed, and how to interpret them. For that purpose we use spectral density analysis (Fig. 15.3, lower part). A spectral

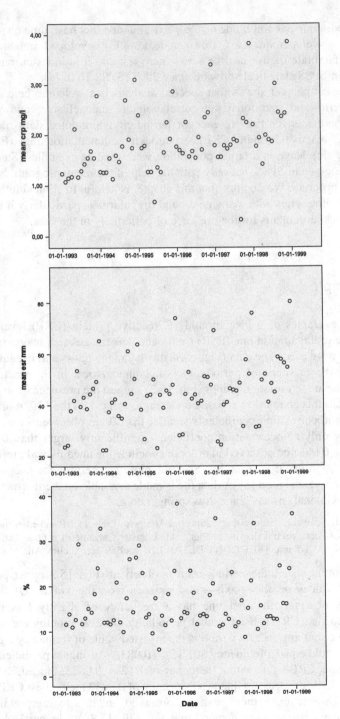

Fig. 15.1 Example of monthly C reactive protein (CRP) levels (mg/l), erythrocyte sedimentation rate (ESR) (mm), and percentages sick leaves (%) in a target population

Fig. 15.2 Autocorrelation coefficients of the date from Fig. 15.1

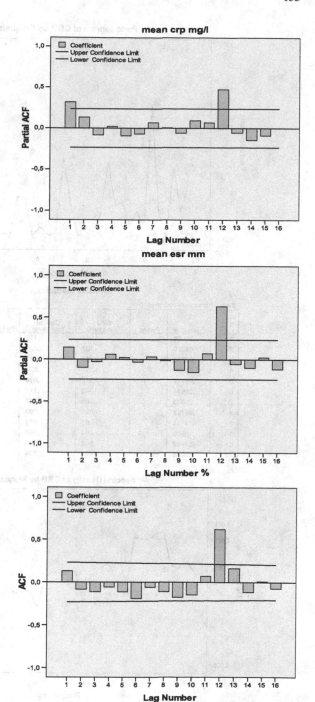

Periodogram of CRP by Frequency

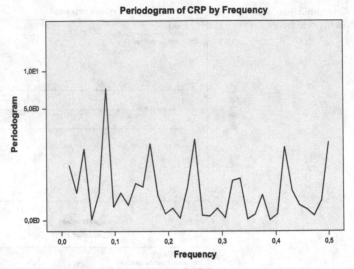

Univariate Statistics

Series Name:mean crp mg/l

	Frequency	Period	Sine Transform	Cosine Transform	Periodogram	Spectral Density Estimate
1	,00000		,000	1,852	,000	8,767
2	,01389		-,197	,020	1,416	12,285
3	,02778		-,123	,012	,552	9,223
4	,04167		-,231	,078	2,144	10,429
5	,05556		,019	,010	,016	23,564
6	,06944		-,040	-,117	,552	22,985
7	,08333		-,365	,267	7,355	19,519
8	,09722		-,057	-,060	,243	20,068
9	,11111		-,101	-,072	,556	20,505
10	,12500		-,004	-,089	,286	5,815
11	,13889		,065	-,135	,811	10,653
12	,15278		-,024	,139	,715	10,559

Spectral Density of CRP by Frequency

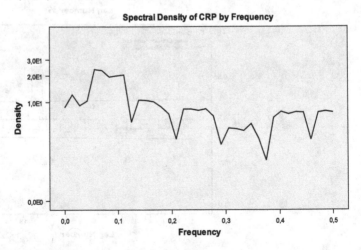

Fig. 15.3 Spectral analysis of the CRP data from Fig. 15.1

density curve is a filtered, otherwise called smoothed, version of the usual periodogram with irregularities beyond a given threshold (noise) filtered out. The spectral density curve of Fig. 15.3 shows five distinct peaks with a rather regular pattern. The lowest frequency simply displays the yearly peak at a frequency of 0.0833. The other peaks at higher frequencies are the result of the Fourier model consistent of sine and cosine functions, and do not indicate additional periodicities. Even so much so that they demonstrate the absence of further periodicities.

The erythrocyte sedimentation rate and % sick leave data of the example can be analyzed with similar command. We should add that the tables of the periodogram data are not displayed if you do not use the paste command which allows you to change syntax rules. The Figs. 15.4 and 15.5 show that, again, an annual periodicity is demonstrated and that, also again, no further periodicities are in the data as demonstrated by the smoothed spectral density curves.

4 Discussion

Seasonal patterns are assumed in many fields of medicine. Examples include the incidence of nosocomial infection in a hospital, seasonal variations in hospital admissions, the course of any disease through time etc. Seasonality is defined as a yearly repetitive pattern of severity or incidence of disease. Seasonality assessments are relevant, since they enable to optimize prevention and therapy. Usually, the mean differences between the data of different seasons or months are used. E.g., the number of hospital admissions in the month of January may be roughly twice that of July. However, biological processes are full of variations and the possibility of chance findings can not be fully ruled out. Autocorrelations [1] can be adequately used for the purpose. It is a technique that cuts time curves into pieces. These pieces are, subsequently, compared with the original data-curve using linear regression analysis. Autocorrelation coefficients significantly different from zero suggest the presence of periodicity. As an example, mean monthly CRP values in a target population can be used (Fig. 15.1, upper part). The data are very peaked and irregular. Figure 15.2 upper part shows the autocorrelation analysis. Although it suggests the presence of seasonality, in all of them this conclusion is based on a single value, i.e., the 12th month value. However, autocorrelation coefficients smaller than 0 are observed in none of the graphs. Not only autocorrelation coefficients significantly larger than 0 but also smaller than 0 must be observed in order to conclude the unequivocal presence of a statistically significant seasonality. Box and Jenkins demonstrated that spectral analysis based on traditional Fourier analyses can be helpful in this situation [3]. First, a Fourier analysis consistent of sine and cosine functions is fitted to the data. Then, an periodogram is computed with outcome values on the y-axis and time frequencies on the x-axis. It displays a peak outcome at the frequency of the expected periodicity (months, years, weeks etc.).

The current chapter shows that spectral analysis can be adequately used with very irregular patterns and inconclusive autocorrelation analysis, and is able to

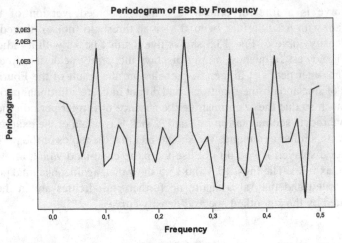

Periodogram of ESR by Frequency

Univariate Statistics

Series Name:mean esr mm

	Frequency	Period	Sine Transform	Cosine Transform	Periodogram	Spectral Density Estimate
1	,00000		,000	44,582	,000	2070,562
2	,01389		-2,270	1,311	247,363	1870,393
3	,02778		-2,133	1,227	218,075	1402,148
4	,04167		-1,829	,432	127,190	1638,481
5	,05556		,981	,071	34,830	4461,648
6	,06944		-1,305	-1,149	108,890	4062,087
7	,08333		-6,485	-,517	1523,774	3863,768
8	,09722		-,437	-,711	25,071	4010,195
9	,11111		-,928	-,263	33,518	3883,374
10	,12500		-,571	-1,619	106,061	545,150
11	,13889		,173	-1,323	64,080	5644,989
12	,15278		-,022	,654	15,397	5741,567

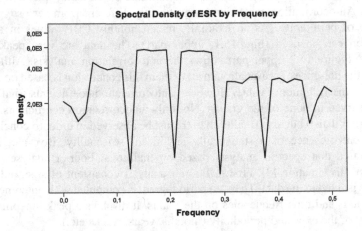

Spectral Density of ESR by Frequency

Fig. 15.4 Spectral analysis of the ESR data from Fig. 15.1

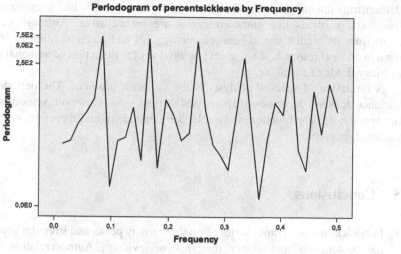

Periodogram of percentsickleave by Frequency

Univariate Statistics

Series Name:%

	Frequency	Period	Sine Transform	Cosine Transform	Periodogram	Spectral Density Estimate
1	,00000		,000	16,884	,000	97,606
2	,01389		,522	,113	10,276	125,210
3	,02778		,261	,506	11,677	184,647
4	,04167		-,725	,380	24,102	327,875
5	,05556		,630	,792	36,906	1956,922
6	,06944		-,405	-1,275	64,422	1947,939
7	,08333		-3,379	3,048	745,586	1924,263
8	,09722		-,128	-,128	1,178	1866,789
9	,11111		-,190	-,538	11,711	1809,789
10	,12500		,004	-,615	13,610	171,055
11	,13889		,579	-,958	45,098	1673,281
12	,15278		-,030	,372	5,005	1667,807

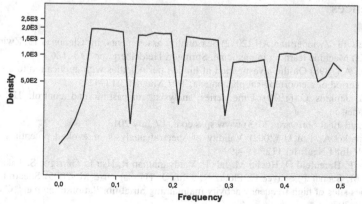

Spectral Density of percentsickleave by Frequency

Fig. 15.5 Spectral analysis of the % sick leave data from Fig. 15.1

demonstrate unequivocal periodicities where visual methods like scatter-grams and traditional methods like autocorrelations are inconclusive. Although currently, apart from its regular use in neurophysiology [5] and electrocardiology [6], little used in clinical research, it has great potential for the detection of seasonal patterns in many fields of medicine.

A limitation of spectral analysis is the variance problem. The periodogram's variance does not decrease with increased sample sizes. However, smoothing using the spectral density function, is sample size dependent, and therefore, reduces the variance problem.

5   Conclusions

1. In clinical research times series often show many peaks and irregular spaces, and the presence of periodicity may not be evident. Autocorrelation analysis reviewed in part one of this three volume edition [1] is helpful, but has a limited sensitivity to detect periodicity.
2. Spectral analysis available in the Forecasting module of SPSS, is based on traditional Fourier analyses, and can be helpful in this situation. It may be more sensitive than autocorrelation analysis.
3. In the examples given, unequivocal periodicities were demonstrated.
4. Smoothed curves obtained from spectral density analysis available in the same module, can demonstrate whether additional period effects do or do not exist.
5. A limitation of spectral analysis is the variance problem. The periodogram's variance does not decrease with increased sample sizes. However, smoothing using the spectral density function, is sample size dependent, and therefore, reduces the variance problem.

References

1. Cleophas TJ, Zwinderman AH (2012) Seasonality assessments. In: Cleophas TJ, Zwinderman AH (eds) Machine learning in medicine. Springer, Heidelberg, pp 113–126
2. Schuster A (1898) On the investigation of hidden periodicities with application to a supposed 26 day period of meteorological phenomena. Terr Magnet 3:13–41
3. Box G, Jenkins G (1970) Time series analysis: forecasting and control. Holden-Day, San Francisco
4. SPSS Statistical Software (2013) www.spss.com. 17 July 2013
5. Kramarenko A, Tan U (2002) Validity of spectral analysis of evoked potentials in brain research. Int J Neurosci 112:489–499
6. Sanders P, Berenfeld O, Hocini M, Jais P, Vaidyanathan R, Hsu L, Garrigue S, Takahashi Y, Rotter M, Sacher F, Scavee C, Ploutz R, Jalife J, Haissaguerre M (2005) Spectral analysis identifies sites of high frequency activity maintaining atrial fibrillation in humans. Circulation 112:789–797

Chapter 16
Newton's Methods

1 Summary

1.1 Background

Regression analyses are commonly used to analyze pharmacodynamic/ -kinetic data. Newton's method is different from traditional regression analysis, because, instead of different parameters for a single function, entirely different functions are compared with one another.

1.2 Objective

To assess the advantages of one method versus the other.

1.3 Methods

Hypothesized examples of dose-effectiveness and a time-concentration studies were analyzed. SPSS statistical software was applied for traditional modeling of linear, quadratic and polynomial functions and Xuru's online Nonlinear Regression Calculator was applied for Newton's regression.

1.4 Results

The best fit Newton's regression produced better or, at least, similar statistics to those of the traditional regression functions (residual sum of squares 0.023 and

T.J. Cleophas and A.H. Zwinderman, *Machine Learning in Medicine: Part Three*, 161
DOI 10.1007/978-94-007-7869-6_16, © Springer Science+Business Media Dordrecht 2013

0.027, P = 0.003 and 0.003). Unlike the traditional functions, the best fit Newton's regression enabled to directly estimate pharmacodynamic/ -kinetic constants, because they were in the form of hyperbolas and exponential functions.

1.5 Conclusions

1. Newton's method is more powerful than traditional regression analysis, because hundreds of mathematical functions, instead of a single one, are checked simultaneously.
2. More power also means that the method does not require large data, like those required for traditional dose-effectiveness and time-concentration studies: n = 15 instead of n > 100 may already produce sensible and significant results.
3. Newton's method is also faster than traditional regression, because it enables to identify the functions' zero values in just a few steps.
4. Newton's method is more complete than traditional regression analysis, because it compares different functions with one another rather than different parameters within a single mathematical function.
5. Newton's method gives the possibility to choose from many functions the ones most convenient to the pathophysiological concepts of the investigator, like the plasma half-life and equations for clearance in drug research.
6. Newton's method is the most advanced way of fitting non-linear data to a mathematical function.

2 Introduction

Traditional regression analysis selects a mathematical function, and, then, uses the data to find the best fit parameters. For example, the parameters a and b for a linear regression function with the equation $y = a + bx$ have to be calculated according to

$$b = \text{regression coefficient} = \frac{\sum (x - \overline{x})(y - \overline{y})}{\sum (x - \overline{x})^2}$$

$$a = \text{intercept} = \overline{y} - b\overline{x}$$

With a quadratic function, $y = a + b_1x + b_2x^2$ (and other functions) the calculations are similar, but more complex. Newton's method works differently [1]. Instead of selecting a mathematical function and using the data for finding the best fit parameter-values, it uses arbitrary parameter-values for a, b_1, b_2, and, then, iteratively measures the distance between the data and the modeled curve until the shortest distance is obtained. Calculations are much more easy than those of traditional regression analysis, making the method, particularly, interesting for comparing multiple functions to one data set.

Isaac Newton, the famous Cambridge UK mathematics professor in 1669, was notoriously reluctant to publish his inventions and his method was first published in 1711 [2]. It was, initially, given little attention, because, at that time, the scientific community was mainly interested in finding the best fit of data to a single function, and was not yet not ready for comparing multiple functions. Only in 1963, with the advent of the computer, computationally intensive methods for comparing multiple functions became possible, and Donald Marquardt, statistician at Dupont, Wilmington, USA, developed a software program including the most common and interesting functions and using Newton's method for analysis [3]. It is now often called non-linear regression or non-linear least squares, and it is available in SPSS (since version 9, 1998) [4] and Excel as an add-on module (XLSTAT_PRO) [5], and widely used, particularly, in physics [6], geometry [7], chemistry [8], biology [9, 10], and econo-/sociometry [11]. However, in clinical research it is little used. Searching Medline we found one HIV-dynamics paper [12], one imaging paper of breast cancer [13], one theoretical molecular pharmacology paper [14], but, otherwise, no clinical pharmacology papers.

The current paper using hypothesized examples of dose-effectiveness and a time-concentration studies assesses the performance of Newton's method. We compare the novel method with traditional regression models.

3 Some Theory

Just like traditional regression analysis Newton's method determines the best fit values of the parameters a, b_1, b_2 for the data given. Both methods used the so-called least squares for the purpose. If the y values of each data point are called the y_{values} and the y values of the function's curve are called y_{curve}, then the goal is to minimize the so-called *residual sum of squares* function:

$$SS = sum\ (y_{data} - y_{curve})^2.$$

Because the "smallest SS for the data" is used as criterion for best fit of the data to the function's curve, the method is called the least squares method. This method is only valid with Gaussian distributions of uncertainty, but in biology this is a common assumption. In order to establish a best fit more accurately and rapidly than traditional regression analysis does, Newton's method is helpful. It is explained in Fig. 16.1. Four tangential lines to a non-linear curve are drawn. The left tangential line crosses the non-linear curve. Here a new tangential is drawn. This one crosses the x-axis, and at this point a new tangential is drawn. This is repeated and soon a tangential is established that crosses the x-axis at y = 0 (the

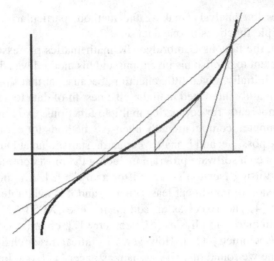

Fig. 16.1 Newton's method: four tangential lines to a non-linear curve are drawn. The left tangential line crosses the non-linear curve. Here a new tangential is drawn. This one crosses the x-axis, and at this point a new tangential is drawn. This is repeated and soon a tangential is established that crosses the x-axis at y = 0 (the root of the function). Only four iterations were required to find the root (zero-point) of this non-linear function. Mathematically, each iteration can be described as: $x_{n+1} = x_n - fx_n/f'x_n$, where $f'x_n$ is the first derivative of fx

root of the function). Only four iterations were required to find the root (zero-point) of this non-linear function. Mathematically, each iteration can be described as:

$$x_{n+1} = x_n - f\,x_n/f'x_n, \text{where } f'x_n \text{ is the first derivative of fx.}$$

An appropriate software program including the most common and interesting functions is now required, and for each of these functions the best fit parameters a, b_1, b_2 etc. are calculated. The magnitude of the residual sum of squares SS is used as criterion for level of fit. Finally, of all best fit functions the one with the smallest overall SS is identified as the ultimately best function for the given data. This method should be more powerful than traditional regression methods, because, instead of a single function, hundreds of them are checked simultaneously.

4 Methods and Results

4.1 Dose-Effectiveness Study

Table 16.1 gives the data of a dose-effectiveness study. Using the commands Analyze, Regression, Curve Estimation, we use SPSS statistical software to draw and calculate the best fit traditional regression equations for a linear, logarithmic,

Table 16.1 Data of dose-effectiveness study

Alfentanil dose x-axis mg/m^2	Effectiveness y-axis [1- pain scale]
0,10	0,1701
0,20	0,2009
0,30	0,2709
0,40	0,2648
0,50	0,3013
0,60	0,4278
0,70	0,3466
0,80	0,2663
0,90	0,3201
1,00	0,4140
1,10	0,3677
1,20	0,3476
1,30	0,3656
1,40	0,3879
1,50	0,3649

quadratic and cubic (polynomial) regression model. Figure 16.2 shows the graphs and Table 16.2 gives the residual sum of squares and the ANOVA (analysis of variance) P-values. All of the models produce a significant fit: the data are closer to the lines than could happen by chance. However, there is a lot of spread in the data. The smallest SS is obtained by the polynomial model. Subsequently a non-linear regression using Newton's algorithm is performed. Although it is available in SPSS [4] and an Excel add-on [5], the easiest way was to use the online Nonlinear Regression Calculator of Xuru's website [15]. This website is made available by Xuru, the world largest business network based in Auckland CA, USA. We simply copy or paste the data of Table 16.1 into the spreadsheet given be the website, then click "allow comma as decimal separator" and click "calculate". Within a few seconds the results come up (Table 16.3). Since Newton's method can be applied to any function, most computer programs fit a given dataset to over 100 functions including Gaussians, sigmoids, ratios, sinusoids etc. For the data given 18 significantly (P < 0.05) fitting non-linear functions were found, the first 6 of them are shown in the Table 16.3. The first one gives the best fit. Its SS is 0.023, equal to that of the cubic function (Table 16.2).

It is the function of a hyperbola:

$$y = 0.42 \ x/(x + 0.17).$$

This is convenient, because, dose-effectiveness curves are, often, successfully assessed with hyperbolas mimicking the Michaelis-Menten equation. The parameters of the equation can be readily interpreted as effectiveness$_{maximum}$ = 0.42, and dissociation constant = 0.17. It is usually very laborious to obtain these parameters from traditional regression modeling of the quantal effect histograms and cumulative histograms requiring data samples of at least 100 or so to be meaningful [16].

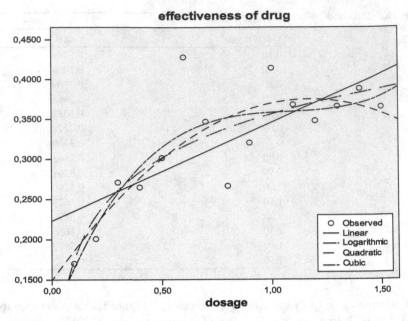

Fig. 16.2 SPSS graph of the linear, logarithmic, quadratic and polynomial (3rd order) models of the dose-effectiveness data from Table 16.1 (x-axis: mg/m^2, y-axis: [1- pain scale])

Table 16.2 Residual sum of squares of standard regression models of the data from Table 16.1

	Non-linear function	Residual sum of squares	P-value
1. Linear	$y = a + bx$	0.036	0.002
2. Logarithmic	$y = a + b \log x$	0.025	0.0001
3. Quadratic	$y = a + b_1x + b_2x^2$	0.025	0.001
4. Polynomial	$y = a + b_1x + b_2x^2 + b_3x^3$	0.023	0.003

Table 16.3 Non-linear functions fitted by Newton's method to the data from Table 16.1

	Non-linear function	Residual sum of squares	P value
1.	$y = 0.42x/(x + 0.17)$	0.023	0.003
2.	$y = -1/(38.4x + 1)^{0.12} + 1$	0.024	0.003
3.	$y = 0.08 \ln x + 0.36$	0.025	0.004
4.	$y = 0.40 e^{-0.11/x}$	0.025	0.004
5.	$y = 0.36x^{0.26}$	0.027	0.004
6.	$y = -0.024/x + 0.37$	0.029	0.005

Figure 16.3 shows an Excel graph of the hyperbolic function fitted to the data. Also, a cubic spline curve going smoothly through every point is drawn. It can be considered as a perfect fit curve. However, unlike Newton's fitted curve, the cubic spline is not accurate for making predictions from the data, because for one segment

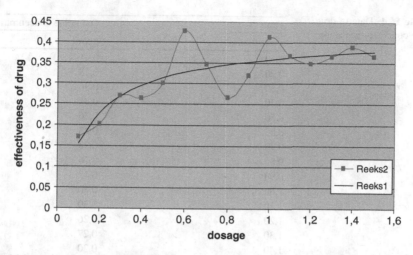

Fig. 16.3 Excel graph of fitted non-linear function to the data of Table 16.1 (x-axis: mg/m^2, y-axis: [1- pain scale]), using Newton's method (the best fit curve is here a hyperbola). A cubic spline goes smoothly through every point, and does this by ensuring that the first and second derivatives of the segments match those that are adjacent

multiple cubic splines (third order polynomial curves) are possible. It can be observed from the figure that the hyperbolic function curve matches the cubic spline curve pretty well.

4.2   Time-Concentration Study

Table 16.4 gives the data of a time-concentration study. Using again the commands Analyze, Regression, Curve Estimation, we use SPSS statistical software to draw and calculate the best fit traditional regression equations for a linear, logarithmic, quadratic and cubic (polynomial) regression model. Figure 16.4 shows the graphs and Table 16.5 gives the residual sum of squares and the ANOVA (analysis of variance) P-values. Again all of the models produce a significant fit: the data are closer to the lines than could happen by chance. However, there is a lot of spread in the data. The smallest SS is again obtained by the polynomial model, but the other models also perform pretty well with very significant p-values. Subsequently a non-linear regression using Newton's algorithm is performed. We use the online Nonlinear Regression Calculator of Xuru's website [15]. We copy or paste the data of Table 16.4 into the spreadsheet, then click "allow comma as decimal separator" and click "calculate". Within a few seconds the results come up. For the data given ten statistically significantly (P < 0.05) fitting non-linear functions were found and shown. For further assessment of the data an exponential function, which is among

Table 16.4 Data of drug time-concentration study

Time	Quinidine concentration
x-axis hours	µg/ml
0,10	0,41
0,20	0,38
0,30	0,36
0,40	0,34
0,50	0,36
0,60	0,23
0,70	0,28
0,80	0,26
0,90	0,17
1,00	0,30
1,10	0,30
1,20	0,26
1,30	0,27
1,40	0,20
1,50	0,17

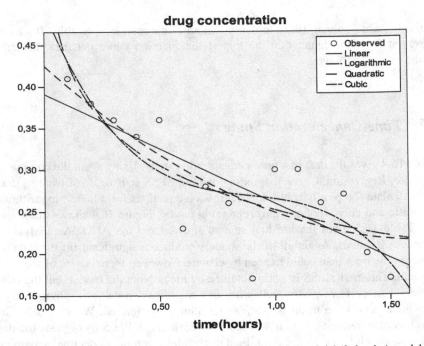

Fig. 16.4 SPSS graph of the linear, logarithmic, quadratic and polynomial (3rd order) models of the dose-effectiveness data from Table 16.5 (x-axis: hours, y-axis: µg/ml)

Table 16.5 Residual sum of squares of standard regression models of the data from Table 16.4

	Non-linear function	Residual sum of squares	P-value
1. Linear	$y = a + bx$	0.029	0.0001
2. Logarithmic	$y = a + b \log x$	0.026	0.0001
3. Quadratic	$y = a + b_1x + b_2x^2$	0.027	0.002
4. Polynomial	$y = a + b_1x + b_2x^2 + b_3x^3$	0.023	0.003

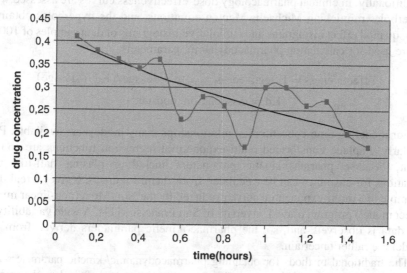

Fig. 16.5 Excel graph of fitted non-linear function to the data of Table 16.5 (x-axis: hours, y-axis: µg/ml), using Newton's method (the best fit curve is here an exponential curve). A cubic spline goes smoothly through every point, and does this by ensuring that the first and second derivatives of the segments match those that are adjacent

the first five shown by the software, is chosen, because relevant pharmacokinetic parameters can be conveniently calculated from it:

$$y = 0.41 \ e^{-0.48 \ x}.$$

This function's SS value is 0.027, which is slightly larger than that of the best traditional regression function (the polynomial function, Table 16.5), but the p-value is still very small and virtually the same (P = 0.003). The following pharmacokinetic parameters are derived:

$$0.41 = C_0 = (\text{administration dosage drug})/(\text{distribution volume})$$

$$-0.48 = \text{elimination constant.}$$

Figure 16.5 shows an Excel graph of the exponential function fitted to the data. Also, a cubic spline curve going smoothly through every point and to be considered as a perfect fit curve is again given. It can be observed from the figure that the exponential function curve matches the cubic spline curve well.

5 Discussion

Traditionally, in clinical pharmacology dose-effectiveness curves are assessed with hyperbolas mimicking Michaelis-Menten equations, and the hyperbolas obtained from quantal effect histograms and cumulative histograms of data samples of 100 or so are used for calculating pharmacodynamic parameters.

$$\text{Effectiveness} = \text{Effectiveness}_{\text{maximum}} \times \text{dosage}/(\text{Kd} + \text{dosage})$$

$$(\text{Kd} = \text{dissociation constant})$$

For modeling time-concentration relationships many models are available. Particularly, Laplace transformed multi-exponential regression functions are convenient, because pharmacokinetic parameters including plasma half-life and equations for clearance can be calculated from them. Figure 16.6 gives a real data example of a multi-exponential curve produced by the Non-Mem (non-linear mixed effect model) program of the University of San Francisco [17]. A wide variability in the data is observed, and, so, the pharmacokinetic parameters derived from the model are rather uncertain.

The traditional methods for obtaining pharmacodynamic/-kinetic parameters are, thus, laborious, and, in addition, due to the generally wide spread of the data, the amount of uncertainty is huge. All of the methods are based on traditional regression modeling to find the best fit regression equation. It means that with help of the data the best fit parameters of various mathematical models are calculated. Newton's method works differently. Instead of different a and b values, different mathematical functions are compared with one another. The current paper suggests that this has many advantages.

Newton's method is, probably, more powerful than traditional regression analysis, because, instead of a single one, hundreds of mathematical functions are checked simultaneously. More power also means that the method does not require large data, like those required for traditional dose-effectiveness and time-concentration studies: n = 15 instead of >100 may already produce sensible and significant results. Newton's method is also faster than traditional regression, because it enables to identify the functions' zero values in just a few steps. Newton's method is more complete than traditional regression analysis, because it compares different functions with one another rather than different parameters within a single mathematical function. Finally, Newton's method gives the possibility to choose from many functions the ones most convenient to pathophysiological concepts, like the plasma half-life and equations for clearance in drug research.

Like traditional regression analyses, Newton's method is a least squares method, and its limitations are similar to the ones of traditional regression. E.g., functions

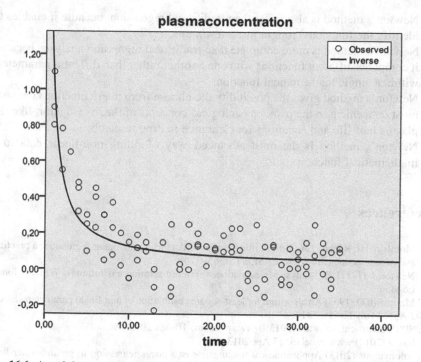

Fig. 16.6 A real data example (x-axis: days, y-axis: μg/ml) of a multi-exponential curve of the time concentration relationship of the long-acting bisphosphonate zolidronine acid produced by Non-Mem regression analysis [17]

may not be obtained or may not be statistically significant with too many outliers in the data, and with overtly non-Gaussian patterns in the data. Like with traditional regression it is meaningful that the investigator has an intuitive feel about the functions established, and about pathophysiological concepts being in agreement with the functions. Nonlinear data are commonly observed in clinical pharmacology. We recommend that the new method be more frequently used in the analysis of real data in clinical research.

6 Conclusions

1. Newton's method is more powerful than traditional regression analysis, because, instead of a single one, hundreds of mathematical functions are checked simultaneously.
2. More power also means that the method does not require large data, like those required for traditional dose-effectiveness and time-concentration studies: n = 15 instead of n > 100 may already produce sensible and significant results.

3. Newton's method is also faster than traditional regression, because it enables to identify the functions' root in just a few steps.
4. Newton's method is more complete than traditional regression analysis, because it compares different functions with one another rather than different parameters within a single mathematical function.
5. Newton's method gives the possibility the choose from many functions the ones most convenient to the pathophysiological concepts of the investigator, like the plasma half-life and equations for clearance in drug research.
6. Newton's method is the most advanced way of fitting non-linear data to a mathematical function.

References

1. Motulsky HJ, Ransna LA (1987) Fitting curves to data using nonlinear regression: a practical and nonmathematical review. FASEB J 1:365–374
2. Newton I (1711) De analysi per aequationes numero terminorum infinitas. William Jones, London
3. Marquardt D (1963) An algorithm for least-squares estimation of non-linear parameters. SIAM J Appl Math 11:431–441
4. SPSS Statistical Software (2013) www.spss.com. 10 Apr 2013
5. Excel (2013) www.excel.nl. 15 Apr 2013
6. Anonymous (2013) Applications of nonlinear least squares regression to ground-water flow modeling, West Central Florida, US Geological Society report 00-4094. fl.water.usgs.gov/PDF. 10 Apr 2013
7. Le Botlan D, Rugraff Y, Ouguerzan L (1996) 180° Pulse imperfection effects on fitting of relaxation curves obtained by low field NMR spectroscopy. Spectrosc Lett 29:1091–1102
8. De Diego A, Madariago J, Chapola E (1997) Effect of additional hydrofluoric acid on the conductivity of concentrated fluorosilicic acid aquous solutions. J Chem Eng Data 42:209–213
9. Corley R, Murphy M (2004) An in vitro technique for measuring the production rate of volatile fatty acids in the rumes under dynamic conditions. Small Rum Res 54:219–225
10. Utomo HD, Hunter KA (2010) Particle concentration adsorption of divalent metal ions on coffee grounds. Bioresour Technol 101:1482–1486
11. Maddala CS (2008) Nonlinear least squares regression. In: Introduction to econometrics, 3rd edn. Wiley, New York
12. Chen J, Wu H (2008) Efficient local estimation for time-varying coefficients in deterministic dynamic models with application to HIV-dynamics. J Am Stat Assoc 103:369–383
13. Yang G, Hipwell JH, Hawkes DJ, Arridge SR (2012) A nonlinear least squares model for solving the joint reconstruction and registration problem of digital breast tomosynthesis. In: Proceedings of medical image understanding and analysis. Department of Computer Science, Swansea University, Swansea, pp 87–92
14. Kemmer G, Keller S (2010) Nonlinear least-squares data fitting in excel spreadsheets. Nat Protoc 5:267–281
15. Online nonlinear regression (2013) http://www.xuru.org/rt/NLR.asp. 4 Sept 2013
16. Brody TM (1994) Concentration-response relationships. In: Brody TM, Larner J, Minneman KP, Neu HC (eds) Human pharmacology, 2nd edn. Mosby, St. Louis, pp 25–32
17. Boeckman AJ, Sheiner LB, Beal SL (1992) NONMEM user's guide of the NONMEM Project Group, University California, San Francisco

Chapter 17
Stochastic Processes: Stationary Markov Chains

1 Summary

1.1 Background

Stationary Markov processes are exponential regression models for guessing the chance of a predicted outcome.

1.2 Objective

To assess how it works and what limitations must be accounted.

1.3 Methods and Results

Patients with diabetes II and beta cell failure, patients at risk of overweight, and a hypothetical example of a population with given genotype frequencies of the alleles A and a were used.

1.4 Results

The stationary Markov models, if correct, would allow for conclusions like:
(a) if beta cell failure occurs in 10 % of the diabetics per year, then in 6.58 years 50 % will have it; (b) if in a population the chances of thin, normal, and overweight

T.J. Cleophas and A.H. Zwinderman, *Machine Learning in Medicine: Part Three*, DOI 10.1007/978-94-007-7869-6_17, © Springer Science+Business Media Dordrecht 2013

sons and fathers are known, then the chance of a thin grandson for a normal granddad can be computed; (c) genotype frequencies of offspring will remain unchanged in future generations (Hardy-Weinberg principle).

1.5   Conclusions

1. Stationary Markov processes are exponential regression models for obtaining a glimpse of the future.
2. Unfortunately, they are very speculative, particularly with humans, because humans continually change their lifestyles.
3. The stationary Markov models, if correct, would allow for computing the chance of beta cell failure after several years, the chance of an overweight grandson, and other exponential time series.

2   Introduction

Stochastic is the Greek adjective for guessing. A stochastic process is a process that assesses or guesses the chance of a predicted outcome. The term was invented by the Russian Mathematician Andrey Markov, a professor of mathematics at the Saint Petersburg University, Russia, 1856–1922 [1]. It is a process for making predictions about the future from the present time. What is special about Markov's stochastic process, is, that its outcome is only determined by its current state, and, that it is independent of its past or future. Markov processes are related to regression modeling. Regression models try to fit experimental data in a mathematical model, e.g., a linear or exponential (logistic and Cox), and, subsequently, test how far distant the data are from the model. Logistic regression assess the odds of an event, Cox regression the hazard of death. Markov models assess the time to a complication or death dependent on the initial state of the underlying disease. Regression models are only valid within the range of the x-values observed. Markov modeling goes one step further, and aims at predicting outside the range of x-values. E.g., it may take years before a complication will take place. Like with logistic and Cox regression Markov models assume an exponential-pattern in the data which may be a strong assumption, because biological processes are full of variations and will not allow for a perfect fit. This is even more a problem, if you want to make predictions outside the range of observations. Markov processes are, therefore, more at risk of unrealistic results than traditional regression modeling. As an example, many conclusions from the Framingham studies [2] were based on Markov processes. Subsequent research has demonstrated that some of the Framingham results were true, some, however, were not [2]. This is probably because patients tend to improve their lifestyle, and new and better treatments have been implemented. Nonetheless, Markov processes have been central to probability assessments not only in fields like socio- and econometry [3], but also in medical science [4].

The current chapter uses examples to review simple two-state Markov chains, as well as stationary Markov chains. It is also demonstrated that the Hardy-Weinberg principle [5] stating that allele and genotype frequencies will remained constant over the generations can be explained as a Markov process.

3 Simple Two-State Markov Chains

3.1 Example 1

As an example, in patients with diabetes mellitus type II, sulfonureas are highly efficacious, but they will, eventually, induce beta-cell failure. Beta-cell failure is sometimes defined as a fasting plasma glucose >7.0 mmol/l. The 1st question is, does the severity of diabetes and/or the potency of the sulfonurea-compound influence the induction of beta-cell failure?

This was studied in 500 patients with diabetes type II.

at time 0 year   0/500 patients   had beta − cell failure
at time 1 year   50/500 patients(= 10 %)   had beta − cell failure

As after 1 year 90 % had no beta-cell failure, it is appropriate according to the Markow model to extrapolate:

after 2 years 90 % × 90 %   = 81 % no beta − cell failure
after 3 years 90 % × 90 % × 90 %   = 73 % no beta − cell failure

How long will it take for 50 % of the patients to have beta-cell failure?

$0.9^x = 0.5$

xlog 0.9 = log 0.5

x = log 0.5/log 0.9 = 6.579

After 6.58 years, 50 % has(no)beta − cell failure.

3.2 Example 2

A 2nd question was, does the severity of diabetes mellitus type II influence induction of beta-cell failure. A cut-off level for severity often applied is a fasting plasma glucose >10 mmol/l. According to the Markov modeling approach the question can be answered as follows:

250 patients had fasting plasma glucose < 10 mmol/l at diagnosis(Group − 1)
250 patients had fasting plasma glucose > 10 mmol/l at diagnosis(Group − 2)

If after 1 year sulfonureas (su) treatment 10/250 of the patients from Group-1 had b-cell failure, and 40/250 of the patients from Group-2, which is significantly different by $p < 0.01$, then we can again extrapolate.

$$(240/250)^x = 0.5$$
$$x \ \log(240/250) = \log \ 0.5$$
$$x = \log \ 0.5/\log \ 0.96 = 16.979$$

In Group-1 it takes 16.98 years before 50 % of the patients developed beta-cell failure.

$$(210/250)^x = 0.5$$
$$x\log(210/250) = \log \ 0.5$$
$$x = \log \ 0.5/\log \ 0.84 = 3.976$$

In Group-2 it takes 3.98 years before 4 % of the patients developed beta-cell failure.

3.3   Example 3

The 3rd question is, does potency of su-compound influence induction of b-cell failure?

250 patients started on amaryl(potent sulfonurea)at diagnosis $(Group - A)$
250 patients started on artosin(non-potent sulfonurea)at diagnosis$(Group - B)$

If after 1 year 25/250 of Group-A had beta-cell failure, and 25/250 of the group-B, it is appropriate according to the Markov model to conclude that a non-potent does not prevent beta-cell failure. Note Markov modeling is highly speculative, because nature does not routinely follow mathematical models.

4   Stationary Markov Chains

4.1   Example 1, Prediction of Coronary Risk Factors

As an example in a study of coronary risk factors in men, fathers' weights were assumed to be a major predictor of the sons' weights. In a population of 10,000 fathers and their sons the weights of fathers and sons were split into three categories, and the proportions of both fathers and sons were calculated. The underneath matrix gives the results. In Markov terms this matrix is called a *Transition matrix.*

	thin (son)	normal	overweight
thin (father)	0.320	0.500	0.180
normal	0.210	0.590	0.200
overweight	0.120	0.480	0.400

From the above transition matrix the underneath chances can be calculated.

What is chance of a normal father to have a thin son 0.210
....normal son 0.590
....overweight son 0.200

What is the chance of a thin father to have a thin son 0.320
....normal son 0.500
....overweight son 0.180

What is the chance of an overweight father to have a thin son 0.120
....normal son 0.480
....overweight son 0.400

Under the assumption that the chances to be observed in the next generation will be the same, the grandsons' data can be predicted by multiplying the chances of the sons with those of the grandsons.

What is chance of a normal father to have a thin grandson?

$$
0.210 \times \begin{array}{l} - \ 0.320 \\ - \ 0.500 \\ - \ 0.180 \end{array} = 0.067
$$

$$
0.590 \times \begin{array}{l} - \ 0.210 \\ - \ 0.590 \\ - \ 0.200 \end{array} = 0.124
$$

$$
0.200 \times \begin{array}{l} - \ 0.120 \\ - \ 0.480 \\ - \ 0.400 \end{array} = 0.024
$$

$$
\underline{} +
$$
$$
0.215
$$

The chance of a normal father to have a thin grandson equals 0.215. If you want to calculate the chances of all of the possible combinations of various categories between granddads and grandson, it will take a lot of pocket calculator computing. However, a matrix pocket calculator can do the job rapidly. Using Bluebit Matrix Calculator freely available on the Internet [6] we were able to multiplicate entire matrices.

Enter the original transition matrix (here we will call it P) into the field under "Enter Matrix A", and copy and paste the same matrix into the field under "enter

Matrix B". Click "Multiply A*B". A Results page comes up showing the expected proportions of the three categories of weight in the grandsons for each granddad category separately. It can be observed that the proportion of thin grandsons for the normal granddads equals 0.215.

$P^2 =$	thin	normal	overweight
thin	0.229	0.541	0.230
normal	0.215	0.549	0.236
overweight	0.187	0.535	0.278

Also the expected weights for the other two classes of granddads can be observed. By multiplying this result one more time with the original data, the expected estimates for the next generation of sons is observed. The results are shown underneath. E.g., a thin father has a 0.214 chance that has grand-grandson is also thin.

$P^3 =$	thin	normal	overweight
thin	0.214	0.544	0.242
normal	0.212	0.545	0.243
overweight	0.205	0.542	0.252

All of the above computations are only true if we assume that the outcome has a strictly exponential relationship with the input (the present state).

The above matrices tell us something about the transition from fathers to sons and grandsons, but nothing about the frequency distribution of the weight categories in the original population of fathers.

Let us assume we have the underneath frequency distribution of the current population of fathers.

thin	normal	overweight
0:200	0:560	0:240

What is chance of thin sons from this population of fathers using the transition matrix pattern as given above?

$$
0.200 \times \begin{array}{l} - \quad 0.320 \\ - \quad 0.500 \\ - \quad 0.180 \end{array} = 0.064
$$

$$
0.560 \times \begin{array}{l} - \quad 0.210 \\ - \quad 0.590 \\ - \quad 0.200 \end{array} = 0.118
$$

$$
0.240 \times \begin{array}{l} - \quad 0.120 \\ - \quad 0.480 \\ - \quad 0.400 \end{array} = 0.050
$$

$$
+ \quad 0.232
$$

The chance of a normal father to have a thin grandson equals 0.232.

It is less laborious to compute this result from the multiplication of the probability matrix of the current population, here commonly called the probability vector, with the transition matrix.

$$[0.200 \quad 0.560 \quad 0.240] * [\text{original transition matrix}]$$
$$* \text{ is signal of multiplication.}$$

For that purpose enter the probability vector into the field "Enter Matrix A", and the original transition matrix into the field under "enter Matrix B". Click "Multiply A*B". The Results page comes up showing the underneath.

$$0.210 \quad 0.546 \quad 0.244.$$

The proportions of the thin, normal and overweight sons are not very different from those of the fathers. We wish to estimate the proportions of the grandsons, and grand-grandsons, and multiply for that purpose the original probability vector with the transition matrices P^2 and P^3.

For that purpose the data of the field "enter Matrix B" is replaced with the data of P^2 and P^3, using the commands cut and paste.

$$0.211 \quad 0.544 \quad 0.245$$
$$0.211 \quad 0.544 \quad 0.245$$

As observed above, the proportions of the grandsons and grand-grandsons are entirely similar to the proportions of the sons. If you would continue a couple of generations, then the results would remain the same. This indicates that on the long-term the frequency distribution of the males is constant, and that it does not depend on the initial distribution of the weight categories, but rather on the pattern of the transition matrix. This observation is relevant in clinical settings, because it enables to make long term predictions about populations.

4.2   Example 2, Hardy-Weinberg Principle

The Hardy-Weinberg principle [5] states that allele and genotype frequencies will remain constant over the generations under the provision that no mutations, ecological disasters and other unexpected events occur. Let us assume in a very simple situation that a population consists of a pool of A and a alleles, and that the alleles A is present in 40 % and a in 60 % of the cases. The underneath matrix shows the possible contributions of father and mothers to the offspring's genotype. Three genotypes are possible.

		males	
		A	a
females	A	AA	Aa
	a	aA	aa

The chance of offspring with AA equals $40\ \% \times 40\% = 16\ \%$.
....aa equals $60\ \% \times 60\ \% = 36\ \%$
......................................Aa equals $60\ \% \times 40\ \% = 24\ \%$
......................................aA equals $40\ \% \times 60\ \% = 24\ \%$

100 randomly selected children of this offspring will provide

$$16 + 16 + 24 + 24 = 80 \text{ A alleles.}$$
and
$$24 + 24 + 36 + 36 = 120 \text{ a alleles.}$$
The ratio $A/a = 80/120 = 40/60 = 40\ \%/60\ \%$.

This means that the allele frequencies of the offspring are the same as those of the parents, and following the same procedure they will stay so for the generations to come.

5   Discussion

Markov's stochastic processes do have major limitations. Unlike regression modeling, they predict beyond the interval of observation, a very hazardous activity, particularly with humans who continually change their life styles. Indeed, the Framingham results have been demonstrated to overestimate the effects of risk factors on cardiovascular disease [2]. Obviously, publications and health measures have reduced the magnitudes of several risk factors. And so do improved treatments and new insights.

Nonetheless, Markov processes show, what would have happened, if not such health measures had been taken. Exponential patterns are accepted bases for many physical and biological processes, like drug elimination kinetics, and radioactivity decline. Logistic and Cox proportional hazard regression are also exponential models, and adequately predicted the chance of clinical events or the time to hazardous events, although mostly within the time of observation. With Markov modeling results outside of the observed values are predicted, and, therefore, they are rather speculative. They are, however fascinating, not for confirmational, but rather for explorative purposes. Mankind is nowadays more interested in its future than it was in the past [7], and much of current machine learning methods is aiming at making such predictions. No method more directly addresses the question "don't you like to see the future sometimes" than the Markov's stochastic processes do, despite their limitations.

6 Conclusions

1. Stationary Markov processes are exponential regression models for obtaining a glimpse of the future.
2. Unfortunately, they are very speculative, particularly with humans, because they continually change their lifestyles.
3. The stationary Markov models, if correct, would allow for conclusions like:

(a) if beta cell failure occurs in 10 % of the diabetics per year, then in 6.58 years 50 % will have it; (b) if in a population the chances of thin, normal, and overweight son and fathers are known, then the chance of a thin grandson for a normal granddad can be computed; (c) if mutations, recombinations and selections are not taken into account, genotype frequencies of offspring will remain unchanged in future generations (Hardy-Weinberg principle).

References

1. Markov AA (1971) Extension of the limit theorem of probability theory to a sum of variables connected in a chain. In: Howard RA (ed) Dynamic probabilistic systems, vol 1: Markov Chains. Wiley, London
2. Brindle P, Emberson J, Lampe F (2003) Predictive accuracy of the Framingham coronary risk score in British men. BMJ 327:1267–1273
3. Durrett R (2010) Probability, theory and examples. Cambridge University Press, Cambridge
4. Fang J, Caixia L (2003) Stochastic processes and their applications in medical science. In: Lu Y, Fang JQ (eds) Advanced medical statistics. World Scientific, River Edge
5. Anonymous (2013) Hardy-Weinberg principle. Wikipedia.org/wiki/Hardy%E2%89%93Weinberg_principle. 8 May 2013
6. Online Matrix Calculator-Bluebit Software (2013) www.bluebit.gr/matrix-c. 8 May 2013
7. Ward P (2008) The future of mankind – how will evolution change humans. Scientific American, New York, NY, USA, 7 December

Chapter 18
Stochastic Processes: Absorbing Markov Chains

1 Summary

1.1 Background

Absorbing Markov chains are used for analyzing irreversible complications, and they are more complex to analyze than stationary Markov chains (Chap. 17), and require higher order matrices.

1.2 Objective

To assess whether non-mathematicians are able to perform analyses.

1.3 Methods

Hypothesized examples of 3 and 4 disease states, like stable (1) coronary artery disease, (2)complications,(3) recovery state, (4) death are used. Bluebit electronic matrix calculators from the internet were used for analyses.

1.4 Results

The chances of a person in state 1 ending up in state 2 or 3 can be computed by a pocket calculator. With larger matrices the electronic matrix calculator readily provides the risk values.

T.J. Cleophas and A.H. Zwinderman, *Machine Learning in Medicine: Part Three*,
DOI 10.1007/978-94-007-7869-6_18, © Springer Science+Business Media Dordrecht 2013

1.5   Conclusions

1. Absorbing Markov chains can be used to analyze the long-term risks of irreversible complications and death.
2. The future is not shown, but it is shown, what will happen, if everything remains the same.
3. Absorbing Markov chains assume, that the chance of an event is not independent, but depends on events in the past.
4. Absorbing Markov chains require higher power matrix algebra, but user friendly electronic matrix calculators are freely available on the internet, and they are easy to use even for non-mathematicians.

2   Introduction

A stochastic process is a mathematical model that evolves over time in a probabilistic way [1]. The term was invented by Andrey Markov, a professor of mathematics at the Saint Petersburg University, Russia, 1856–1922 [2]. Markov processes are related to regression modeling. Regression models try to fit experimental data in a mathematical model, e.g., a linear or exponential (logistic and Cox), and, subsequently, test how far distant the data are from the model. Regression models are only valid within the range of the x-values observed. Markov modeling is also exponential but goes one step further. It aims at predicting outside the range of x-values. It assumes, e.g., that per time unit the same percentage of patients has stable disease, and a stable risk profile. The unstable patients, however, generally have a larger risk which may get better, if they recover, or not, if they do not. It is possible to construct a matrix of risks and predict the time to events and other complications from it for entire populations and individuals with a particular risk profile. Matrices in which patients ultimately recover are called regular or stationary. However, in clinical research most matrices involve irreversible complications and death, and such matrices are more complex to analyze. They are called absorbing matrices, with the irreversible complications called the absorbing states of the patients [3].

Absorbing Markov chains have been applied for making long-term predictions from population surveys like National Health Surveys and cohort studies like the Framingham studies [4]. We believe that even if the predicted results of this research did often not precisely match the data ultimately observed [5, 6], because of better treatments and lifestyles changing risk patterns, the methodology is worthwhile, because it demonstrates future risks based on knowledge of today, and should, therefore, be a motivation for further improvements.

Absorbing matrices can not be analyzed without the help of some matrix algebra, and this paper will give some step by step analyses of real data examples. It was particularly written for clinical investigators who are not familiar with matrix algebra and are willing to accept some steps intuitively and without mathematical proof. The "fundamental matrix" method recommended by Charles Grinstead, mathematician at Swarthmore College Philadelphia, PE, USA, in 1996, will be used [7]. The online Bluebit Matrix calculator is applied for computations [8].

3 Regular and Irregular Markov Chains

As an example, in patients with diabetes mellitus type II, sulfonureas are highly efficacious, but they will, eventually, induce beta-cell failure. Beta-cell failure is sometimes defined as a fasting plasma glucose >7.0 mmol/l. The 1st question is, does the severity of diabetes and/or the potency of the sulfonurea-compound influence the induction of beta-cell failure? This was studied in 500 patients with diabetes type II.

at time 0 year   0/500 patients   had beta-cell failure
at time 1 year   50/500 patients (= 10 %)   had beta-cell failure.

As after 1 year 90 % had no beta-cell failure, it is appropriate according to the Markow model to extrapolate:

after 2 years 90 % × 90%   = 81 % no beta-cell failure
after 3 years 90 % × 90 % × 90%   = 73 % no beta-cell failure

How long will it take for 50 % of the patients to have beta-cell failure?

$0.9^x = 0.5$
$x \log 0.9 = \log 0.5$
$x = \log 0.5 / \log 0.9 = 6.579$
After 6.58 years   = 50 % no beta-cell failure.

In clinical research patients are often classified into multiple subgroups with different chances, and it is impossible to calculate exact prognoses of the subgroups without the use of some matrix algebra. The above example can also be analyzed using the underneath matrix.

	At time 1 year Chance of no beta cell failure	yes beta cell failure
At time 0 year		
If you had no beta cell failure	[0.9	0.1]
If you had beta cell failure	[0.0	1.0]

This 2×2 matrix (M) must be multiplied by the 0 year data pattern (= 100 % no beta cell failure) to produce the percentages after 1 year. The percentages after subsequent years is obtained by multiplying the 0 year data pattern with M^2, M^3, M^4, etc. The following percentages are obtained.

	Percentages no beta cell failure	beta cell failure
1 year	90 %	10 %
2	81	19
3	72.9	27.1
4	65.6	34.4
5	59.0	41.0
6	53.1	46.9
7	47.8	52.2

The result is identical to that of the initial computation. Approximately halfway between the 6th and seventh year 50 % of the patients will have beta-cell failure. It is obvious that, ultimately, virtually all of the patients will have beta-cell failure. The situation would be different if some of the beta cell failure patients would recover. An equilibrium would develop with similar numbers of patients turning from one category into the other. This equilibrium would e.g. be 50/50 % with the underneath matrix.

	At time 1 year Chance of no beta cell failure	yes beta cell failure
At time 0 year		
If you had no beta cell failure	[0.9	0.1]
If you had beta cell failure	[0.1	0.9]

Markov chains with some of the patients ultimately going into an irreversible stage are called absorbing or irregular Markov chains, while those with an equilibrium are called regular or stationary Markov chains.

4   Example 1

Patients with three states of treatment for a disease are checked every 4 months. The underneath matrix is a so-called transition matrix. The states 1–3 indicate the chances of treatment: 1 = no treatment, 2 = surgery, 3 = medicine. If you are in state 1 today, there will be a $0.3 = 30$ % chance that you will receive no treatment in the next 4 months, a $0.2 = 20$ % chance of surgery, and a $0.5 = 50$ % chance of medicine treatment. If you are still in state 1 (no treatment) after 4 months, there will again be a 0.3 chance that this will be the same in the second 4 month period etc. So, after 5 periods the chance of being in state 1 equals $0.3 \times 0.3 \times 0.3 \times 0.3 \times 0.3 = 0.00243$. The chance that you will be in the states 2 or 3 is much larger, and there is something special about these states. Once you are in these states you will never leave these chance-states anymore, because the patients who were treated with either surgery or medicine are no longer followed in this study. That this happens can be observed from the matrix: if you are in state 2 at one time, you will have a chance of $1 = 100$ % to stay in state 2 and chance $0 = 0$ % not to do so. The same is true for the state 3.

	State in next period (4 months)		
	1	2	3
State in current time			
1	0.3	0.2	0.5
2	0	1	0
3	0	0	1

Now we will compute what will happen with the chances of a patient in the state 1 after several 4 month periods.

	chances of being in a state		
	state 1	state 2	state 3
4 month period			
1st	30 %	20 %	50 %
2nd	$30 \times 0.3 = 9$ %	$20 + 0.3 \times 20 = 26$ %	$50 + 0.3 \times 50 = 65$ %
3rd	$9 \times 0.3 = 3$ %	$26 + 9 \times 0.2 = 27.8$ %	$65 + 9 \times 0.5 = 69.5$ %
4th	$3 \times 0.3 = 0.9$ %	$27.8 + 3 \times 0.2 = 28.4$ %	$69.5 + 3 \times 0.5 = 71.0$ %
5th	$0.9 \times 0.3 = 0.27$ %	$28.4 + 0.9 \times 0.2 = 28.6$ %	$71.0 + 0.9 \times 0.5 = 71.5.$

Obviously, the chances of being in the states 2 or 3 increase, though increasingly slowly, and the chance of being in state 1 is, ultimately, going to approximate zero. In clinical terms: postponing the treatment does not make much sense, because everyone in the no treatment group will eventually receive a treatment and the ultimate chances of surgery and medicine treatment are approximately 29 and 71 %. With larger matrices this method for calculating the ultimate chances is rather laborious, and, in addition, approximate. Matrix algebra offers a rapid method that is also more exact, instead of approximate. This example is very simple and more complex examples can be solved in the same way.

	State in next period (4 months)			
	1	2	3	
State in current time				
1	[0.3]	[0.2	0.5]	matrix Q matrix R
2	[0]	[1	0]	matrix O matrix I
3	[0]	[0	1]	

First, the states are called transient, if they can change (the state 1), and absorbing if not (the states 2 and 3). Then, the original matrix is partitioned into four submatrices, otherwise called its canonical form:

[0.3]	Upper left corner.
	This square matrix Q can be sometimes very large with rows and columns respectively presenting the transient states.
[0.2 0.5]	The upper right corner.
	This R matrix presents in rows the chance of being absorbed from the transient state.
[1 0]	The lower right corner.

(continued)

(continued)

[0 1]	This identity matrix I presents rows and columns with chances of being in the absorbing states, the I matrix must be adjusted to the size of the Q matrix (here it will look like (1) instead of [1 0].

$$[0 \quad 1]$$

[0]	The lower left corner.
[0]	This is a matrix of zeros (0 matrix).

From the above matrices a so-called fundamental matrix (F) is constructed.

$$[(\text{ matrix I }) \quad - \quad (\text{ matrix R })]^{-1} \quad = [0.7]^{-1} = 10/7$$

With larger matrices a matrix calculator, like the Bluebit Online Matrix Calculator [8] can be used to compute the matrix to the -1 power by clicking "Inverse".

The fundamental matrix F equals 10/7. It can be interpreted as the average period of time, before someone goes into the absorbing state ($10/7 \times 4$ months $= 5.714$ months). The product of the fundamental matrix F and the R matrix gives more exact chances of a person in state 1 ending up in the states 2 and 3.

$$F \times R = (10/7) \times [0.2 \quad 0.5] = [2/7 \quad 5/7] = [0.285714 \quad 0.714286].$$

The two values add up to 1.00, which indicates a chance of ending up in one of the two absorbing states equal to 100 %.

5   Example 2

Patients with three states of treatment for a chronic disease are checked every 4 months.

	State in next period (4 months)		
	1	2	3
State in current time			
1	0.3	0.6	0.1
2	0.45	0.5	0.05
3	0	0	1

The above matrix of three states and second periods of time gives again the chances of different treatment for a particular disease, but it is slightly different from the above one. Here state 1 = no treatment state, state 2 = medicine treatment, state 3 = surgery state. In the example we assume that medicine can be stopped while surgery is irretrievable, and, thus, an absorbing state. We first partition the matrix.

	State in next period (4 months)				
	1	2	3		
State in current time					
1	[0.3	0.6]	[0.1]	matrix Q	matrix R
2	[0.45	0.5]	[0.05]		
3	[0 0]		[1]	matrix O	matrix I

The R matrix	$[0.1 \ ]$ $[0.05 \ ]$	is in the upper right corner.
The Q matrix	$[0.3 \ \ 0.6 \ ]$ $[0.45 \ \ 0.5 \ ]$	is in the left upper corner.
The I matrix	$[1]$	is in the lower right corner, and must be adjusted, before it can be subtracted from the Q matrix according to $\begin{bmatrix} 1 & 0 \\ 0 & 1 \end{bmatrix}$.
The 0 matrix	$[0 \ \ 0]$	is in the lower left corner.

$$I - Q = \begin{bmatrix} 1 & 0 \\ 0 & 1 \end{bmatrix} - \begin{bmatrix} 0.3 & 0.6 \\ 0.45 & 0.5 \end{bmatrix} = \begin{bmatrix} 0.7 & -0.6 \\ -0.45 & 0.5 \end{bmatrix}$$

The inverse of $[I - Q]$ is obtained by marking "Inverse" at the online Bluebit Matrix Calculator [8] and equals

$$[I - Q]^{-1} = \begin{bmatrix} 6.25 & 7.5 \\ 5.625 & 8.75 \end{bmatrix} = \text{fundamental matrix F.}$$

It is interpreted as the average periods of time before some transient state goes into the absorbing state ($(6.25 + 7.5 = 13.75) \times 4$ months for the patients in state 1 first and state 2 second and $(5.625 + 8.75 = 14.375) \times 4$ months for the patients in state 2 first and state 1 second).

Finally, the product of matrix F times matrix R is calculated. It gives the chances of ending up into the absorbing state for those starting in the states 1 and 2.

$$\begin{bmatrix} 6.25 & 7.5 \\ 5.625 & 8.75 \end{bmatrix} \times \begin{bmatrix} 0.1 \\ 0.05 \end{bmatrix} = \begin{bmatrix} 1.00 \\ 1.00 \end{bmatrix}$$

Obviously the chance of both the transient states for ending up in the absorbing state is $1.00 = 100\%$.

6 Example 3

State 1 = stable coronary artery disease (CAD), state 2 = complications, 3 = recovery state, 4 = death state).

	State in next period (4 months)			
	1	2	3	4
State in current time				
1	0.95	0.04	0	0.01
2	0	0	0.9	0.1
3	0	0.3	0.3	0.4
4	0	0	0	1

If you take higher powers of this transition matrix (P), you will observe long-term trends of this model. For that purpose use the matrix calculator and square the transition matrix (P^2 gives the chances in the 2nd 4 month period etc.) and compute also higher powers (P^3, P^4, P^5, etc.).

P^2
0.903 0.038 0.036 0.024
0.000 0.270 0.270 0.460
0.000 0.090 0.360 0.550
0.000 0.000 0.000 1.000
P^6
0.698 0.048 0.063 0.191
0.000 0.026 0.064 0.910
0.000 0.021 0.047 0.931
0.000 0.000 0.000 1.000

The above higher order transition matrices suggest that with rising powers, and, thus, after multiple 4 month periods, there is a general trend towards the absorbing state: in each row the state 4 value continually rises. In the end we all will die, but in order to be more specific about the periods of time involved in this process, a special matrix procedure like the one described in the previous examples is required. In order to calculate the precise time before the transient states go into the absorbing state, we need to partition the initial transition matrix.

	State in next period (4 months)						
	1	2	3		4		
State in current time							
1	[0.95	0.04	0	]	[0.01]		
2	[0	0	0.9	]	[0.1]	matrix Q	matrix R
3	[0	0.3	0.3	]	[0.4]		
4	[0	0	0	]	[1]	matrix O	matrix I

$$F = (I - Q)^{-1}$$

$$I - Q = \begin{bmatrix} 1 & 0 & 0 \\ 0 & 1 & 0 \\ 0 & 0 & 1 \end{bmatrix} - \begin{bmatrix} 0.95 & 0.04 & 0.0 \\ 0.0 & 0.0 & 0.9 \\ 0.0 & 0.3 & 0.3 \end{bmatrix}$$

$$F = \begin{bmatrix} 0.05 & -0.04 & 0 \\ 0.0 & 1.0 & -0.9 \\ 0.0 & -0.3 & 0.7 \end{bmatrix}^{-1}$$

The online Bluebit Matrix calculator, marking inverse, produces the underneath result.

$$F = \begin{bmatrix} 20.0 & 1.302 & 1.674 \\ 0.0 & 1.628 & 2.093 \\ 0.0 & 0.698 & 2.326 \end{bmatrix}$$

The average time before various transient states turn into the absorbing state (dying in this example) is given.

State 1 : $(20 + 1.302 + 1.674) \times 4$ months $= 91.904$ months.
State 2 : $(0.0 + 1.628 + 2.093) \times 4$ months $= 14.884$ months.
State 3 : $(0.0 + 0.698 + 2.326) \times 4$ months $= 12.098$ months.

The chance of dying for each state is computed from matrix F times matrix R (click multiplication, enter the data in the appropriate fields and click calculate.

$$FR = \begin{bmatrix} 20.0 & 1.302 & 1.674 \\ 0.0 & 1.628 & 2.093 \\ 0.0 & 0.698 & 2.326 \end{bmatrix} \times \begin{bmatrix} 0.01 \\ 0.1 \\ 0.4 \end{bmatrix} = \begin{bmatrix} 1.0 \\ 1.0 \\ 1.0 \end{bmatrix}$$

Like in the previous examples again the products of the matrices F and R show that all of the states end up with death. However, in the state 1 this takes much more time than it does in the other two states.

7 Discussion

Only discrete time Markov chains are reviewed. However, using the time as a continuous variable is possible. It does, though, require a more complex approach, and various differential equations have to be applied [6].

Markov chains have been criticized for making inadequate predictions [4, 5]. However, the goal is not to show the future as something unavoidable, but rather to demonstrate, based on current information, what will happen, if everything remains the same.

Another point about Markov chains is that it is assumed to be an entirely new way of probabilistic thinking in science [9, 10]. Until Markov's lecture in Jan 1913 [10], a century ago, the scientists thought that series of events were generally independent of one another.

Markov proposed the concept of interdependence of events. In contrast with probability explained with numbers of coin flippings, as a set of mutually independent observations, it might be better to have it explained with a game like monopoly: moves rely on a roll of the dice, but where the player ends also depends on where he/she began. Suddenly, the probability where to end was linked to the probability where to start. This approach has fundamentally changed the way we think about life and about science in particular. This was recently summarized by Gordon Ireland in the Harvard Gazette [10].

In the past few years Markov chain technology has found new applications. It has been implemented in decision trees for modeling the prognosis of patients subsequent to the choice of particular management strategies [11]. Simulated cohorts and Monte Carlo simulations are used for the purpose [12]. Also medical cost-effectiveness analyses made use of this technology [12]. Markov chains have been used in life sciences e.g. for assessing immune response in rabbits, and behavior patterns in mice [1]. It was applied for evaluating hospital admission rates [13], medical record analyses, like bed planning and resource allocation research [14]. It has been used in the field of medical imaging [15], and epidemiological modeling like disease dynamics [16].

The current chapter explains absorbing Markov chains as a straightforward method to compute the expected time to complications, death and other events in clinical research that can be performed by clinical investigators with little mathematical background on the provision that an electronic matrix calculator is used.

8 Conclusions

1. Absorbing Markov chains are used to analyze the long-term risks of irreversible complications and death.
2. The future is not shown, but it is shown, what will happen, if everything remains the same.
3. Absorbing Markov chains assume, that the chance of an event is not independent, but depends on events in the past.
4. Absorbing Markov chains require higher power matrix algebra, but user-friendly electronic matrix calculators are freely available on the internet, and they are easy to use even for non-mathematicians.

References

1. Anonymous (2013) Markov Chains, think about it. Addison Wesley product. Pearson Education Inc. www.pearsoned.com. 29 May 2013
2. Markov AA (1971) Extension of the limit theorem of probability theory to a sum of variables connected in a chain. In: Howard R (ed) Dynamic probabilistic systems, vol 1: Markov Chains, Wiley, London
3. Mentch L (2013) Absorbing Markov chains. www.facstaff.bucknell.edu/ap030/Math3451. 30 May 2013
4. Brindle P, Emberson J, Lampe F (2003) Predictive accuracy of the Framingham coronary risk score in British men. BMJ 327:1267–1273
5. Durrett R (2010) Probability, theory and examples. Cambridge University Press, Cambridge
6. Fang J, Caixia L (2003) Stochastic processes and their applications in medical science. Chapter 26. In: Lu Y, Fang JQ (eds) Advanced medical statistics. World Scientific, River Edge, pp 991–1032
7. Grinstead CM, Snell JL (1997) Introduction to probability. AMS Bookstore, Philadelphia
8. Online Matrix Calculator – Bluebit Software (2013) www.bluebit.gr/matrix-c. 8 May 2013
9. Ward P (2008) The future of mankind-how will evolution change humans. Scientific American, 7 December
10. Ireland G (2013) An idea that changed the world. Harvard Gazette, the official organ of the Harvard University, Cambridge, 29 May 2013, pp 1–5
11. Sonnenberg FA, Beck JB (1993) Markov models in medical decision making: a practical guide. Med Decis Making 13:322–328
12. Hazen G (2012) Markov versus medical Markov modeling. Powerpoint presentation. Northwestern University, Chicago, February 2012
13. Bartolomeo N, Trerotoli P, Moretti A, Serio G (2008) A Markov model to evaluate hospital readmission. BMC Res Methodol 8:23–26
14. Liu CH, Wang KM, Guh YY (1991) A Markov chain model for medical record analysis. J Oper Res Soc 42:357–364
15. Kupinski MA, Hoppin JW, Clarkson E, Barrett HH (2003) Ideal-observer computation in medical imaging with use of Markov chain Monte Carlo techniques. J Oper Soc Am Opt Image Sci Vis 20:430–438
16. Zipkin EF, Christopher SJ, Cooch EG (2010) A primer on the application of Markov chains to the study of wildlife disease dynamics. Meth Ecol Evol 1:192–198

Chapter 19
Conjoint Analysis

1 Summary

1.1 Background

Conjoint analysis determines how people value different characteristics of a product.

1.2 Objective

To assess whether this methodology can be applied in clinical research.

1.3 Methods

A simulated data example of 15 physicians expressing their preferences for a novel medicine was used. SPSS statistical software was applied for data analysis.

1.4 Results

Safety and price were the most important characteristics with correlation coefficients between the observed preferences computed from the physicians' data and the prediction model constructed by the conjoint module of 0.988 and 0.931 (both $p < 0.0001$). The Kendall's test for holdouts showed that the chance of absence of a type I error was 75.02 %, suggesting a moderate validity of the model.

T.J. Cleophas and A.H. Zwinderman, *Machine Learning in Medicine: Part Three*,   195
DOI 10.1007/978-94-007-7869-6_19, © Springer Science+Business Media Dordrecht 2013

1.5   Conclusions

1. Conjoint analysis answers questions like what is important to clients, who plan to book a flight, buy a car or any other product.
2. Not only in marketing research but also in medicine conjoint analysis may be relevant for the assessment of choices made by the consumers rather than the producers of a product.
3. Advantages include: (1) psychological effects are important and are included in consumer decisions; (2) the best fit overall preference level to a medicine with a specified pattern enables to make predictions about any future medicine; (3) the selected preferences give information about the interactions between different characteristics.
4. Disadvantages include: (1) it is pretty complex; (2) it may be hard to respondents to express preferences; (3) other characteristics not selected may be important too, e.g., physical and pharmacological factors.
5. Conjoint analysis is a wonderful method because it assesses what is really important to patients/doctors.

2   Introduction

Conjoint analysis was invented by Paul Green, a professor of mathematical psychology at Cornell University, Ithaca, New York, USA, in the 1980s [1]. It determines how people value different features (attributes, aspects, characteristics, factors) of a product or service. It answers questions like what is important to clients, who plan to book a flight, buy a car, or any other product. Often choices are made by trading off perceived advantages against disadvantages. For example, a low price and a high quality will be most likely be prefered to a high price and low quality, but other characteristics like color and size may play a role too. With conjoint analysis first a limited number of important characteristics of a product like a car is selected by the investigator, and each characteristic is given a level, e.g., from cheap to very expensive etc. Then, orthogonal modeling of the characteristics is performed. Orthogonal modeling is a principle of many multidimensional regression models. Orthogonality in a multiple linear regression analysis means that a predictor variable and his outcome variable are in a single two-dimensional plane, and any other predictor variable is in a plane that is orthogonal with the first plane [2]. The correlation level between the two predictors are zero. It means they are independent of one another and their covariance does, thus, not have to be taken into account. This largely facilitates the computations of standard errors and further analysis of the data. Orthogonal modeling is also applied in machine learning methods like factor analysis [2], partial least squares [3], and discriminant analysis [4].

Conjoint analysis, although already commonly used in marketing research [5], and available in SPSS statistical software [3], is rarely used in medical research. When searching Medline, except for a single pharmaceutical proceedings paper [6], we found no publication. However, the physicians' preferences for choosing a medicine may be just as important to a pharmaceutical company or health institute, as the clients' preferences for booking a flight to an airliner is. This point was recently emphasized in a Wikipedia paper [7].

In the current chapter, using a simulated example of 15 physicians' preferences listings for a medicine with a number of characteristics, we will explain conjoint analysis for the medical research community. SPSS statistical software will be used [8], and stepwise analyses will be given for the benefit of readers who wish to apply this wonderful new methodology that assesses choices made by the consumers rather than the producers of a product.

3 Example, Constructing an Orthogonal Design and Analysis Plan

We want to assess the physicians' judgments about the properties (characteristics, features etc.) of a novel medicine important to their patients. The physicians are requested to judge five characteristics: (1) safety expressed in three levels, (2) efficacy in 3, (3) price in 3, (4) pill size in 2, and prolonged activity in 2 levels. Five characteristics with 2 and 3 levels will theoretically produce $3 \times 3 \times 3 \times 2 \times 2 = 108$ combinations, and this number is, obviously, too large for patients '/physicians' meaningful judgments. In addition, some combinations (in conjoint analysis often called profiles, e.g., a high price and low efficacy will never be prefered and could be skipped from the listing of alternative profiles. The solution is orthogonal modeling of a limited but representative number of profiles. SPSS statistical software is used for the purpose.

> Command: Data. . ..Orthogonal Design. . ..Generate. . ..Factor Name: enter safety. . ..Factor Label: enter safety design. . ..click Add. . ..click ?. . ..click Define Values: enter 1,2,3 on the left, and A,B,C on the right side. . ..Do the same for all of the characteristics (here called factors). . ..click Create a new dataset. . ..Dataset name: enter medicine_plan. . ..click Options: Minimum number of cases: enter 18. . ..mark Number of holdout cases: enter 4. . ..Continue. . ..OK.

The output sheets show a listing of 22 instead of 108 (combinations) profiles with two new variables (status_ and card_) A representative orthogonal selection of the 108 profiles is given by the profiles 1–18 (status_= Design). All of the levels of the different characteristics are equally frequently present, e.g., the safety levels 1,2,3 are observed 6 times each, the pillsize level 1,2 are observed nine times each. Four additional profiles are given by the software program, the holdout cases (status_= Holdout). They will not be used for data analyses but rather for checking the validity of the orthogonal program performed. For further use of the model designed of a physicians' survey, we will first need to perform the Display Design commands.

Command: Data....Orthogonal Design....Display....Factors: transfer all of the characteristics to this window....click Listing for experimenter....click OK.

The output sheet shows a plan card, which looks virtually the same as the above 22 profile listing. The orthogonal design must be saved. E.g., use the name medicine_plan.sav for the purpose. For convenience the orthogonal design is given at "chap19medicine_plan.sav" on the internet at extras.springer.com. The next thing is to use SPSS' syntax program for a conjoint program for our plan.

4 Example, Constructing a Conjoint.sps File

The next thing is to use SPSS' syntax program for a conjoint program for our plan.

Command: click File....move to Open....move to Syntax....enter the following text....
CONJOINT PLAN='g:medicine_plan.sav'
/DATA='g:medicine_prefs.sav'
/SEQUENCE=PREF1 TO PREF22
/SUBJECT=ID
/FACTORS=SAFETY EFFICACY (DISCRETE)
PRICE (LINEAR LESS)
PILLSIZE PROLONGEDACTIVITY (LINEAR MORE)
/PRINT=SUMMARYONLY.
Save this syntax file at the directory of your choice.

Note: the conjoint file entitled CONJOINT.sps does only work, if both the plan file and the data file are correctly entered in the above text. In our example we saved both files at a USB stick (recognised by our computer under the directory "g:"). For convenience the conjoint file entitled "chap19CONJOINT.sps" is also given at extras.springer.com. Prior to use it should be saved at the same USB-stick.

5 Example, Constructing an Experimental Data File and Performing the Conjoint Analysis

The 22 profiles produced by the orthogonal design can now be used to perform an conjoint analysis with real data. For that purpose 15 physicians were requested to express their preferences of the 22 different profiles. The data are entered in an SPSS file with the IDs (the individual numbers given to the physicians) and the 22 profiles as variables (the columns), and the individual physicians as rows. The data file entitled "chap19medicine_prefs.sav" is given on the internet at extras.springer.com. The conjoint analysis of the experimental data is now performed.

> Command: click CONJOINT.sps....the above syntax text is shown....click Run...select All.

6 Example, the Output of the Conjoint Analysis

The output sheets are subsequently given by the program. Table 19.1 gives an overview of the different characteristics (here called factors), and their levels used to construct an orthogonal design and analysis plan of the data from our example. Table 19.2 gives the utility scores, which are the overall levels of the preferences expressed by the physicians requested what is important to them while choosing a medicine for their patient. The meaning of the levels are given:

safety level B: best safety
efficacy level A: best efficacy
pill size 2: smallest pill
prolonged activity 2: prolonged activity present
price $8: most expensive pill.

Generally, higher scores mean greater preference. There is an inverse relationship between pill size and preference, and between pill costs and preference. There is a negative relationship between pill cost and preference. The safest pill and the most efficaceous pill were given the best preferences. However, the regression coefficients for efficacy were not statistically very significant, and, therefore this predictors of preference was not very large, and could as well be a chance finding. Nonetheless, they were included in the overall analysis by the software program. As the utility scores are simply linear regression coefficients of a multiple linear model, the scores can be used to compute total utilities (add-up preference scores) for a product with known characteristics (feature or factor levels). An interesting thing about the methodology is that, like with linear regression modeling, the characteristic levels can be used to calculate an individual add-up utility score (preference score) for a pill with the underneath characteristics:

(1) pill size (small) + (2) prolonged activity (yes) + safety (C) + efficacy (high) + price ($4) = 1.250+0.733+3.850−0.178−1.189+constant (10.328) = 14.974.

Table 19.1 Gives an overview of the different characteristics (here called factors), and their levels used to construct an orthogonal design and analysis plan of the data from our example	Model description		
		N of levels	Relation to ranks or scores
	Safety	3	Discrete
	Efficacy	3	Discrete
	Price	3	Linear (less)
	Pillsizes	2	Discrete
	prolongedactivity	2	Discrete
	All factors are orthogonal		

Table 19.2 Gives the utility scores, which are the overall levels of the preferences expressed by the physicians requested what is important to them while choosing a medicine for their patient

Utilities		Utility estimate	Std. error
safety	A	−2,222	,167
	B	1,878	,167
	C	,344	,167
efficacy	A	,300	,167
	B	−,244	,167
	C	−,056	,167
pillsize	1	−1,250	,125
	2	1,250	,125
prolongedactivity	1	−,733	,125
	2	,733	,125
price	$4	−1,189	,145
	$6	−2,378	,289
	$8	−3,567	,434
(Constant)		12,539	,318

For the underneath pill the add-up utility score is, as expected, considerably lower.

(1) pill size (large) + (2) prolonged activity (no) + safety (A) + efficacy (low) + price ($8) = −1.250−0.733+1.283−0.533−3.567+constant (10.328) = 5.528.

The above procedure is the real power of conjoint analysis. It enables to predict preferences for profiles that were not rated by the physicians. In this way you will obtain an idea about the preference to be received by a medicine with known characteristics.

The Table 19.2 gives the linear regression coefficients for the factors that are specified as linear. Also non-linear regression and discrete regression is possible. The interpretation of the utility (preference) score for the cheapest pill equals $4 times −1.189 = −4.756 (Table 19.3).

Table 19.4 gives the range of the utility (preference) scores for each characteristic (from high to low). It is an indication of how important the characteristic is compared to the overall preferences of a product. Characteristics with greater ranges play a larger role than the others. As observed the safety and price are the most important preference producing characteristics, while prolonged activity, efficacy, and pill size appear to play a minor role according to the respondents' judgments. The ranges are computed such that they add-up to 100 (%).

Table 19.5 gives the correlation coefficients between the observed preferences computed from the preferences as given by the respondents to a selection of profiles and the preferences calculated from the orthogonally modeled conjoint construct. The correlation both by Pearson and Kendall's method is very good, indicating that the conjoint methodology produces sensitive prediction models. The regression analysis of the hold out cases is intended as a validity check, and produces a pretty large p-value of 24.8 %. Still it means that we have about 75 % to find no type I error in this procedure.

Table 19.3 The table gives
the linear regression
coefficients for the factors
that are specified as linear

Coefficients	
	B coefficient
	Estimate
price	−1,189

The interpretation of the utility (preference) score for the cheapest pill equals $4 times −1.189 = −4.756

Table 19.4 The range of the utility (preference) scores for each characteristic (from high to low) is an indication of how important the characteristic is compared to the overall preferences of a product (here a medicine)

Importance values	
safety	35,163
efficacy	14,373
pillsize	13,355
prolongedactivity	10,388
price	26,721

Averaged importance score

Table 19.5 The table shows the correlation coefficients between the observed preferences computed from the preferences as given by the respondents to a selection of profiles and the preferences calculated from the orthogonally modeled conjoint construct

Correlations[a]		
	Value	Sig.
Pearson's R	,988	,000
Kendall's tau	,931	,000
Kendall's tau for Holdouts	,333	,248

[a]Correlations between observed and estimated preferences

Table 19.6 shows that the conjoint program reports the number of physicians whose preference was opposite to what was expected. They are few. Only in the price-characteristic 5 of the 10 physicians chose differently from expected.

7 Discussion

The current chapter shows that not only in marketing research but also in medicine conjoint analysis is relevant for the assessment of choices made by the consumers rather than the producers of a product. Advantages include the following. First, the physicians' choices may be rather subjective, and not only physical effects but also psychological effects play a role. These psychological effects are included in the analysis. Second, the methodology enables to find the best fit overall preference level to a medicine with a specified pattern of characteristic levels, and is therefore suitable to make predictions about future medicines. Third, the selected preferences

Table 19.6 The conjoint program shows the number of physicians who whose preference was opposite to what was expected

Number of reversals			
Factor	price		5
	prolongedactivity		0
	pillsize		0
	efficacy		0
	safety		0
Subject	1	Physician 1	0
	2	Physician 2	0
	3	Physician 3	0
	4	Physician 4	0
	5	Physician 5	1
	6	Physician 6	1
	7	Physician 7	1
	8	Physician 8	0
	9	Physician 9	0
	10	Physician 10	0
	11	Physician 11	1
	12	Physician 12	0
	13	Physician 13	0
	14	Physician 14	0
	15	Physician 15	1

by the physicians give information about the interactions between the different characteristics. The disadvantages include the following. First, it is pretty complex. Multiple files have to be produced before an analysis is possible, and not only menu commands but also syntax commands have to be given. Second, it may be hard to respondents to express preferences. Third, other characteristics not selected by the investigator may be important to the physicians too, e.g., physical and pharmacological factors. Nonetheless conjoint analysis is a wonderful method because it assesses what is really important to patient/doctors.

8   Conclusions

1. Conjoint analysis determines how people value different characteristics of a product, and answers questions like what is important to clients, who plan to book a flight, buy a car or any other product.
2. Not only in marketing research but also in medicine conjoint analysis may be relevant for the assessment of choices made by the consumers rather than the producers of a product.
3. Advantages include: (1) psychological effects are important and are included in consumer decisions; (2) the best fit overall preference level to a medicine with a specified pattern enables to make predictions about any future medicine; (3) the selected preferences give information about the interactions between the different characteristics.

4. Disadvantage include: (1) it is pretty complex; (2) it may be hard to respondents to express preferences; (3) other characteristics not selected may be important too, e.g., physical and pharmacological factors.
5. Conjoint analysis is a wonderful method because it assesses what is really important to patient/doctors.

References

1. Green PE, Srinivasan V (1978) Conjoint analysis in consumer research: issues and outlook. J Consum Res 5:1023–1033
2. Cleophas TJ, Zwinderman AH (2013) Chapter 14 Factor analysis. In: Cleophas TJ, Zwinderman AH (eds) Machine learning in medicine part one. Springer, Heidelberg, pp 167–181
3. Cleophas TJ, Zwinderman AH (2013) Chapter 16 Partial least squares. In: Cleophas TJ, Zwinderman AH (eds) Machine learning in medicine part one. Springer, Heidelberg, pp 197–212
4. Cleophas TJ, Zwinderman AH (2013) Discriminant analysis. In: Cleophas TJ, Zwinderman AH (eds) Machine learning in medicine part one. Springer, Heidelberg, pp 215–224
5. Gustaffson A, Hermann A, Huber F (2001) Conjoint analysis as an instrument of market research practice. In: Conjoint measurement: methods and applications. Springer, Heidelberg, pp 5–46
6. Furlan R, Corradetti R (2006) Aspects of experimental design in the prescription-based conjoint analysis model. In: Sixth proceedings of ENBIS (European Network of Business and Industrial Statistics), Wroclaw, Poland
7. Anonymous (2013) Conjoint analysis (healthcare). http://en.wikipedia.org/Conjoint_analysis_healthcare. 7 July 2013
8. SPSS Statistical Software (2013) www.spss.com. 7 July 2013

Chapter 20
Machine Learning and Unsolved Questions

1 Summary

1.1 Background

Traditional statistical methods are not always able to solve unsolved scientific questions

1.2 Objective

To assess whether machine learning methodologies can be helpful in these situations.

1.3 Methods

A real data example of 2,000 admissions to hospital was studied for the risk of iatrogenic admissions.

1.4 Results

Unlike traditional methods for data analysis (descriptive statistics, logistic regression, and categorical regression), machine learning methodology was able to discover that a large outlier group of all age patients with iatrogenic admissions used exceptionally many co-medications.

T.J. Cleophas and A.H. Zwinderman, *Machine Learning in Medicine: Part Three*,
DOI 10.1007/978-94-007-7869-6_20, © Springer Science+Business Media Dordrecht 2013

1.5   Conclusions

1. Outlier assessment using machine learning methods, despite a lack of mathe-matical definition of the term outliers, is important in therapeutic research, because outliers can lead to catastrophic consequences.
2. Traditional methods for data analysis, like descriptive statistics, logistic and categorical regression analyses, may be unable to demonstrate outliers.
3. Machine learning methods as described here and in the other chapters of this 3 volume book, allow, for the identification of relevant unknown patterns, and many of these machine learning methods are available in SPSS statistical software.
4. Machine learning is helpful to solve unsolved scientific questions.

2   Introduction

Machine learning is different from traditional data analysis, because, unlike means and standard deviations, it uses proximities between data, data patterns, pattern recognition, data thresholding and data trafficking. This might mean that some data files may better fit machine learning methodologies than traditional methods. In the current chapter a real data example of a 2,000 patient study for iatrogenic admis-sions to hospital was used.[1] The major prior hypothesis was that the numbers of co-medications would be a strong determinant of iatrogenic admission. SPSS statistical software was applied [2]. We will show that it is worthwhile in the event of inconclusive traditional analyses to explore the data using machine learn-ing methodologies like cluster analyses. An SPSS data file is provided in extras. springer.com, and step-by-step analyses are described for the benefit of investiga-tors who wish to practice and perform their own analyses.

3   Example, Traditional Analyses

In a 2,000 patient study of hospital admissions 576 possibly iatrogenic were identified by a team of specialists [1]. Table 20.1 gives the patient characteristics. Two thousand admissions to a general hospital were analyzed. Traditional binary logistic regression with the risk of iatrogenic admission as outcome and the vari-ables, age, gender, numbers of co-medications, and numbers of co-morbidities as predictor variables was performed. SPSS was used. The data file is entitled "chap20iatrogenicadmissions.sav", and is available on the internet in extras. springer.com.

Command: Analyze....Regression....Binary Logistic....Dependent: select iatrogeni-cadmission....Covariates: select age, gender, comorbidity, comedication....click OK.

Table 20.1 Characteristics of all admissions assessed (n = 2,000) (24 indications for admission, the indications for admission in >5 % of the cases are shown)

Age (years, mean, SD, range)	69	39	16–88
Gender (males, %)	52.5		
Duration of admission (days, mean, SD)	6.7	7.4	
Mortality (proportion)	0.04		
Admissions through emergency room (number, %, 95 % confidence interval)	1,942	97	96–98
Indications for admission	Number	%	Confidence intervals (95 %)
1. Cardiac condition and hypertension	810	40.5	38.0–42.1
2. Gastrointestinal condition	254	12.7	11.9–14.2
3. Infectious disease	200	10.0	9.2–12.0
4. Pulmonary disease	137	6.9	6.5–7.7
5. Hematological and malignant conditions	183	9.2	6.7–11.1

In the output sheets look at "Variables in equation". The Table 20.2 shows that except for age none of the predictors were significant predictors of the risk of having a iatrogenic admission.

The logistic analysis was based on the assumption that the relationship between the numbers of co-medications and risk of iatrogenic admission would be linear, and this, of course, needs not necessarily be true. Therefore we, subsequently, performed a categorical logistic regression, with the numbers of co-medications assessed as categories instead of increasing quantities.

Command: Analyze....Regression....Binary Logistic....Dependent: select iatrogeni-cadmission....Covariates: select age, gender, comorbidity, comedication....click Categorical....transfer comedications to Categorical Covariates....click Continue.... click OK.

The outcome sheets show the multiple logistic model with co-medications as categorical predictor variable (Table 20.3). The upper part shows the results of the recordings per number of co-medication. The lower part gives a more compact picture of the results. With the four predictor variables now both age and co-medication are very significant predictors at p < 0001 and p = 0.011. However, a categorical analysis is not easy to interpret, because different types of relationships between the categories and the risk of an event (iatrogenic admission) are possible. For that purpose we drew bar charts and computed cross-tabs. SPSS [2] was used again.

Command: Graphs....Legacy Dialog....Bar....click Simple....click Summary for groups of cases....click Define....transfer co- medications to Category Axis....transfer iatrogenic admission to Columns....click OK.

The output sheet gives a bar chart (Fig. 20.1), showing that in the no iatrogenic group indicated by ",00" (n = 1,424) a falling trend in admissions was observed

Table 20.2 Multiple binary regression analysis of 2,000 admissions to hospital with the odds of iatrogenic admission as *dependent* variable and age (variable 1), gender (variable 2), presence of co-morbidity (variable 9, yes = 0, no = 1), and number of co-medications (variable 10, zero to eight co-medications) as *independent* variables (p-values <0.10 are defined statistically significant)

Variables in the equation

	B	S.E.	Wald	df	Sig.	Exp(B)
Step 1[a] age	−,019	,003	29,317	1	,000	,981
gender	,091	,101	,808	1	,369	1,095
comedication	,089	,064	1,958	1	,162	1,093
comorbidity	,085	,065	1,718	1	,190	1,088
Constant	35,174	6,778	26,928	1	,000	1,888E15

[a]Variable(s) entered on step 1: age, gender, comedication, comorbidity

Table 20.3 Co-medication has been recorded from a continuous into a categorical variable with 9 categories (zero to 8 co-medications), (p-values <0.10 are defined statistically significant)

Variables in the equation

	B	S.E.	Wald	df	Sig.	Exp(B)
Step 1[a] age	−,019	,004	28,506	1	,000	,981
gender	,082	,102	,650	1	,420	1,086
comedication			19,843	8	,011	
comedication(1)	19,445	40167,898	,000	1	1,000	2,784E8
comedication(2)	19,990	40167,898	,000	1	1,000	4,805E8
comedication(3)	19,810	40167,898	,000	1	1,000	4,012E8
comedication(4)	20,070	40167,898	,000	1	1,000	5,204E8
comedication(5)	19,538	40167,898	,000	1	1,000	3,056E8
comedication(6)	19,906	40167,898	,000	1	1,000	4,414E8
comedication(7)	19,493	40167,898	,000	1	1,000	2,922E8
comedication(8)	41,474	56823,717	,000	1	,999	1,028E18
comorbidity	,101	,067	2,254	1	,133	1,107
Constant	15,437	40167,898	,000	1	1,000	5062628,819

[a]Variable(s) entered on step 1: age, gender, comedication, comorbidity

Variables in the equation

	B	S.E.	Wald	df	Sig.	Exp(B)
Step 1[a] age	−,019	,004	28,506	1	,000	,981
gender	,082	,102	,650	1	,420	1,086
comedication			19,843	8	,011	
comorbidity	,101	,067	2,254	1	,133	1,107
Constant	15,437	40167,898	,000	1	1,000	5062628,819

[a]Variable(s) entered on step 1: age, gender, comedication, comorbidity

with increasing numbers of co-medications. In the yes iatrogenic admission indicated by "1,00" (n = 576), however, a steady pattern was observed from 0 to 3 co-medications, and, then, the numbers became rather small. A cross-tab was computed.

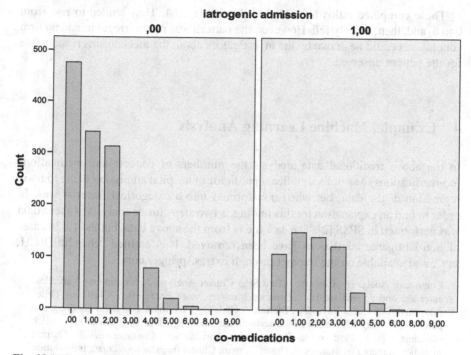

Fig. 20.1 Bar chart, showing that in the no iatrogenic group indicated by ",00" (n = 1,424) a falling trend in admissions was observed with increasing numbers of co-medications. In the yes iatrogenic admission indicated by "1,00" (n = 576), however, a more steady pattern was observed

Table 20.4 The values of the bar charts from Fig. 20.1, and their ratios

iatrogenic admission * co-medications crosstabulation

Count

		Co-medications									
		,00	1,00	2,00	3,00	4,00	5,00	6,00	8,00	9,00	Total
iatrogenic admission	,00	476	341	313	186	79	21	6	0	1	1,423
	1,00	108	150	141	123	35	15	3	1	0	578
Total		584	491	454	309	114	38	9	1	1	1,999

Ratios	0.227	0.440	0.450	0.661	0.443	0.714
0.500	0.000					

Command: Analyze….Descriptive Statistics. …Crosstabs. …transfer iatrogenic admission to Row(s). …transfer co-medications to Column(s). …click OK.

Table 20.4 shows the values of the bar charts from Fig. 20.1, and the odds (the ratios) are calculated according to

$$\frac{\text{iatrogenic admissions}}{\text{no-iatrogenic admissions.}}$$

These computed ratios are added to the Table 20.4. They tended to rise from 0 to 6, and, then, sharply fell. However, the pattern was rather irregular, and no firm conclusions could be drawn by the investigators about the mechanisms responsible for the pattern observed.

4 Example, Machine Learning Analysis

In the above traditional data analysis the numbers of concomitant medications (co-medications) was not a significant predictor of hospital admission in the logistic regression of the data, but when transformed into a categorical factor it was. In order to find an explanation for this finding, a two step cluster analysis of these data was performed in SPSS [2]. The data file is from the above data, but the 1,424 cases of non-iatrogenic admissions have been removed. It is entitled "chap20BIRCH. sav", and available on the internet through extras.springer.com.

> Command: Analyze….Classify….Two Step Cluster Analysis ….Continuous Variables: enter age and co-medications….Distance Measure: mark Euclidean….Clustering Criterion: mark Schwarz's Bayesian Criterion….click Options: mark Use noise handling …. percentage: enter 25….Assumed Standardized: enter age and co-medications….click Continue….click Plot: mark Cluster pie chart….click Continue….click Output: Statistics….mark Descriptives by cluster….mark Cluster frequencies….mark Information Criterion ….Working Data File: mark Create cluster membership variable….click Continue….click OK.

Table 20.5 gives the autoclustering table of the two-step procedure. It can be observed that 15 different models are assessed (including 1–15 clusters). This table shows something about the precision of the different models, as estimated by the overall uncertainties (or standard errors) of the models (measured by Schwarz's Bayesian Criterion (BIC) = n ln (standard error)^2 + k ln n, where n = sample size, ln = natural logarithm, k = number of clusters). With the 3 or 4 cluster models the smallest BIC was observed, and, thus, the mostly precise model. The 3 or 4 cluster model, including an outlier cluster, would, therefore, be an adequate choice for further assessment of the data. The Tables 20.6 and 20.7 gives description and frequency information of the 4 cluster model. Figure 20.2 gives a pie chart of the size of the 3 clusters and the outlier cluster. If we minimize this output page, and return to the data file, we will observe that SPSS [2] has provided again the membership data. This file is too large to understand what is going on, and, therefore we will draw a three dimensional graph of this output.

> Command: Graphs….Legacy Dialogs….3 D Bar Charts….X-axis represents: click Groups of cases….Y- axis represents: click Groups of cases….click Define….Variable: enter co-medications….Bars represent: enter mean of values….X-Category axis: enter age….Y-Category axis: enter two step cluster number variable….click OK.

Figure 20.3 shows the result. In front two clusters with younger patients and few co-medications are observed. In the third row is 1 cluster of elderly with

Table 20.5 15 different cluster models have been assessed by the two-step procedure (including 1–15 clusters)

Auto-clustering

Number of clusters	Schwarz's Bayesian Criterion (BIC)	BIC change[a]	Ratio of BIC changes[b]	Ratio of distance measures[c]
1	293,899			
2	277,319	−16,580	1,000	1,513
3	185,362	−91,957	5,546	1,463
4	178,291	−7,071	,426	1,007
5	197,946	19,654	−1,185	1,141
6	216,403	18,457	−1,113	1,159
7	236,467	20,064	−1,120	1,099
8	251,072	14,606	−,881	1,629
9	272,582	21,509	−1,297	1,125
10	291,641	19,059	−1,150	1,015
11	301,090	9,449	−,570	1,000
12	308,019	6,929	−,418	1,058
13	321,943	13,924	−,840	1,197
14	339,382	17,439	−1,052	1,074
15	361,262	21,880	−1,320	1,225

The precision of the different models, as estimated by the overall uncertainties measured by Schwarz's Bayesian Criterion (BIC) is given. With the 3 or 4 cluster models the smallest BIC was observed, and, thus, the most precise model
[a]The changes are from the previous number of clusters in the table
[b]The ratios of changes are relative to the change for the two cluster solution
[c]The ratios of distance measures are based on the current number of clusters against the previous number of clusters

Table 20.6 Description information of the 4 cluster model selected from the 15 models from Table 20.5

Centroids

		Age		Comed	
		Mean	Std. deviation	Mean	Std. deviation
Cluster	1	1928,9227	6,50936	2,5028	,50138
	2	1933,7171	6,01699	,6250	,48572
	3	1956,8551	6,16984	1,0725	,64895
	Outlier (−1)	1939,7644	20,15623	2,4138	1,75395
	Combined	1936,8090	14,91570	1,8090	1,34681

Table 20.7 Frequency information of the 4 cluster model selected from the 15 models from Table 20.5

Cluster distribution

		N	% of combined	% of total
Cluster	1	181	31,4 %	9,1 %
	2	152	26,4 %	7,6 %
	3	69	12,0 %	3,5 %
	Outlier (−1)	174	30,2 %	8,7 %
	Combined	576	100,0 %	28,8 %
Excluded cases		1,424		71,2 %
Total		2,000		100,0 %

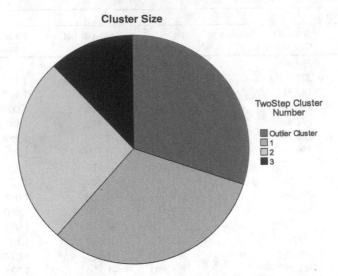

Cluster Size

Fig. 20.2 Pie chart of the cluster size of the 4 cluster model selected from the 15 models from Table 20.5

Fig. 20.3 Three-dimensional bar chart of the 4 cluster model selected from the 15 models from Table 20.5. Over 100 bars indicating mean numbers of co-medications in age classes of 1 year. In the clusters 2 and 3 the patients are young and have few co-medications, in the cluster 1 the patients are old and have many co-medications, in the outlier cluster all ages are present and exceptionally high numbers of co-medications are frequently observed

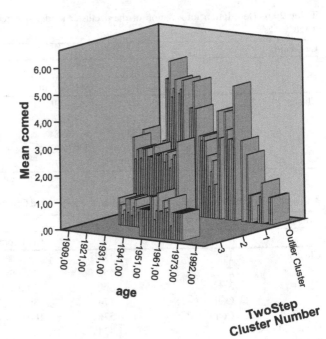

considerably more co-medications. Then, at the back the patients are who do not fit in any of the clusters. They are of all ages, but their numbers of co-medications are generally very high. This finding is relevant, because it supports a deleterious effect of numbers of co-medications on the risk of iatrogenic admission.

5 Discussion

The current chapter shows that in spite of inconclusive descriptive statistics, logistic regressions and categorical regressions, machine learning methodologies were able to provide clinically relevant patterns in the data helpful in clinical practice. Obviously, The young and middle aged persons have few co-medications, the older have many co-medications. However, there is a large outlier category of patients with iatrogenic admissions. They are of all ages and use exceptionally many co-medications. Thus, this is consistent with the concept that many co-medications is a serious risk of iatrogenic admission.

Machine learning often does not offer rigorous mathematical definitions like those for outliers in a dataset, unlike there are for, for example, p-values, r-values etc. Why then worry about the outliers? This is, because they can lead not only to serious misinterpretations of the data, but also to catastrophic consequences once the data are used for making predictions, like serious and, sometimes, even fatal adverse events from drug treatments.

We should add that this clustering method points to remote points in the data and flags them as potential outliers. It does not confirm any other prior expectation about the nature or pattern of the outliers. The outliers, generally, involve both extremely high and extremely low values. The approach is, obviously, explorative, but, as shown in the examples, it can produce interesting findings, and theories, although waiting for confirmation. The current cluster analysis is based on proximities. Other forms of machine learning, using data patterns, pattern recognition, data thresholding, data trafficking, are more suitable still for other types of data. The current book Machine Learning in Medicine Part Three as well as the Parts One and Two of this volume gives examples of many methodologies widely available both in SPSS and other software programs.

More complex data than the current data using two-dimensional cluster analysis are possible, although the computations will rapidly become even more laborious and computer memory may rapidly fall short. In the future this kind of research will be increasingly performed through a network of computer systems rather than a single computer system let alone standalone computers. Also, multidimensional outliers may be harder to interpret, because they are associated with multiple factors.

6   Conclusions

1. Outlier assessment using machine learning methods, despite a lack of mathematical definition of the term outliers, is important in therapeutic research, because outliers can lead to catastrophic consequences.
2. Traditional methods for data analysis, like descriptive statistics, logistic and categorical regression analyses, may be unable to demonstrate outliers.
3. Machine learning methods as described here and in the other chapters of this 3 volume book, allow for the identification of relevant unknown patterns, and many of these machine learning methods are available in SPSS statistical software.

References

1. Atiqi R, Cleophas TJ, Van Bommel E, Zwinderman AH (2010) Prevalence of iatrogenic admissions to the departments of medicine/cardiology/pulmonology in a 1250 beds general hospital. Int J Clin Pharmacol Ther 48:517–521
2. SPSS Statistical Software (2013) www.spss.com. 2 Sept 2013

Index

A

Absorbing Markov chains, 8, 183–192
Absorbing matrices, 184
Absorbing states of patients, 184, 188, 190
Add-up preference scores, 199
Advanced models, 92
Affymetrix exon chips, 11, 13
AICC, 91
Akaike's information criterion (AIC), 77, 91
Alleles, 173
Alpha (α), 23
Alternative hypothesis, 21, 48, 50
Amplitudes, 152
Analysis of covariance, 3
Analysis of variance (ANOVA), 3, 8, 21,
    25–27, 30, 70, 84, 130, 165, 167
Analysis of (co-) variance (AN(C)OVA), 3
Analysis plan, 197–199
Angiotensin II receptor antagonists, 13
Annual periodicity, 152
Anomaly detection, 4
ANOVA. *See* Analysis of variance (ANOVA)
AN(C)OVA. *See* Analysis of (co-) variance
    (AN(C)OVA)
Appropriate weights, 7
Approximate solution, 12
Area under the curve (AUC), 23, 53, 87
ARIMA. *See* Autoregressive integrated
    moving average (ARIMA)
Artificial intelligence, 12
Artificially improved data, 56
Assessment of over-dispersion, 78
Association rule learning, 4
Autocorrelation, 2, 4, 151, 160
Autocorrelation coefficients, 152, 155
Autoregressive integrated moving average
    (ARIMA), 4

B

Bar charts, 207, 209
Basic machine learning methods, 1
Bayesian information criterion (BIC), 77, 91
Bayesian networks, 1, 4, 9, 20, 44
Best fit genes, 12
Best fit linear equations, 138
Best fit mathematical function, 8
Best fit mathematical model, 7
Best fit models, 12
Best fit Newton's regression, 162
Best fit parameter-values, 162
Best fit regression equation, 96
Best fit tree, 139
Beta (β), 23
Bhattacharya modeling, 4
Biased data interpretation, 92
Biases of reported methods, 3
Big data, 2, 5, 7, 20
Big observational data, 6
Binary decision trees, 2
Binary logistic regressions, 63, 65–67, 146
Binary partitioning, 2
Binary variable, 21, 34, 63
Bin models, 41
Binning process, 40, 41
Binning syntax, 38
Bin variable, 42
Biological assays, 65
Biological evolution mechanisms, 11, 12
Biological processes full of variations, 157, 174
Biomarkers, 13
Bivariate probit regression, 66
Black box methods, 106, 112
Bluebit matrix calculator, 185, 191
Bonferroni-correction, 24, 26, 27, 31
Bonferroni test, 19, 26

Printed in the United States
By Bookmasters